RAND NATIONAL DEFENSE RESEARCH INSTITUTE

Delivering Clinical Practice Guideline–Concordant Care for PTSD and Major Depression in Military Treatment Facilities

Kimberly A. Hepner, Coreen Farris, Carrie M. Farmer, Praise O. Iyiewuare, Terri Tanielian, Asa Wilks, Michael Robbins, Susan M. Paddock, Harold Alan Pincus

Prepared for the Defense Centers of Excellence for Psychological Health and Traumatic Brain Injury

Approved for public release; distribution unlimited

For more information on this publication, visit www.rand.org/t/RR1692

Library of Congress Cataloging-in-Publication Data is available for this publication.
ISBN: 978-0-8330-9749-1

Published by the RAND Corporation, Santa Monica, Calif.
© Copyright 2017 RAND Corporation
RAND® is a registered trademark.

Cover: photo by Sgt. Jason Kemp, 1st Infantry Division Headquarters.

Limited Print and Electronic Distribution Rights

This document and trademark(s) contained herein are protected by law. This representation of RAND intellectual property is provided for noncommercial use only. Unauthorized posting of this publication online is prohibited. Permission is given to duplicate this document for personal use only, as long as it is unaltered and complete. Permission is required from RAND to reproduce, or reuse in another form, any of its research documents for commercial use. For information on reprint and linking permissions, please visit www.rand.org/pubs/permissions.

The RAND Corporation is a research organization that develops solutions to public policy challenges to help make communities throughout the world safer and more secure, healthier and more prosperous. RAND is nonprofit, nonpartisan, and committed to the public interest.

RAND's publications do not necessarily reflect the opinions of its research clients and sponsors.

Support RAND
Make a tax-deductible charitable contribution at
www.rand.org/giving/contribute

www.rand.org

Preface

The U.S. Department of Defense (DoD) strives to maintain a physically and psychologically healthy, mission-ready force, and the care provided by the Military Health System (MHS) is critical to meeting this goal. Given the rates of posttraumatic stress disorder (PTSD) and major depressive disorder (MDD) among U.S. service members, attention has been directed to ensuring the quality and availability of programs and services targeting these and other psychological health conditions. Understanding the capacity of the MHS and its providers to deliver high-quality care for PTSD and MDD is an important step in support of future efforts to improve care across the MHS.

DoD's Defense Centers of Excellence for Psychological Health and Traumatic Brain Injury (DCoE) asked the RAND Corporation to conduct an assessment of the capacity of the MHS to deliver evidence-based care for PTSD and MDD and to recommend areas in which the MHS could focus its efforts to continuously improve the quality of care provided to all service members. This document is the final report on the results of that study. Specifically, this report (1) provides an overview of the psychological health (PH) workforce at military treatment facilities (MTFs), (2) describes the extent to which PH providers within MTFs report delivering guideline-concordant care for PTSD and MDD, (3) identifies facilitators and barriers to providing this care, and (4) provides recommendations to increase the use and monitoring of guideline-concordant care for PTSD and MDD. It complements other RAND studies that have examined administrative data and medical records of service members diagnosed with PTSD or depression to assess the types of care they actually received.

This report should be of interest to MHS personnel who provide care for service members with PTSD or depression. It should also be useful to those responsible for improving the quality of such care through a variety of approaches (e.g., provider training, programs to incentivize or encourage improved quality, quality monitoring). Finally, the report should be informative to those who work to enhance the structural capacity to deliver psychological health care within the MHS, including senior leaders at Health Affairs and the Defense Health Agency responsible for health policies that guide MHS providers.

This research was sponsored by DCoE and conducted within the Forces and Resources Policy Center of the RAND National Defense Research Institute, a federally funded research and development center sponsored by the Office of the Secretary of Defense, the Joint Staff, the Unified Combatant Commands, the Navy, the Marine Corps, the defense agencies, and the defense Intelligence Community.

For more information on the RAND Forces and Resources Policy Center, see www.rand.org/nsrd/ndri/centers/frp or contact the director (contact information is provided on the web page).

Contents

Figures

Tables

Summary

Addressing psychological health (PH) conditions among U.S. service members remains a pressing challenge for the U.S. Department of Defense (DoD). The Military Health System (MHS) plays a critical role in maintaining a physically and psychologically healthy, mission-ready force. Ensuring the quality and availability of programs and services targeting two of the most common conditions diagnosed and treated in the MHS—posttraumatic stress disorder (PTSD) and major depressive disorder (MDD)—is a key contributor to this goal.

To provide accessible, high-quality care for PH conditions, the MHS has increased the size of its PH workforce by 34 percent (U.S. Government Accountability Office, 2015), established training programs in evidence-based treatments (Borah et al., 2013; Center for Deployment Psychology, undated), developed innovative programs to address PH needs (Weinick et al., 2011), and implemented other approaches to enhance the availability and quality of PH care. However, it is unclear whether these efforts have resulted in a system of care that meets the needs of service members with PH conditions, and little is known about the facilitators and barriers to delivering high-quality, evidence-based PH care.

To help address these questions, DoD's Defense Centers of Excellence for Psychological Health and Traumatic Brain Injury (DCoE) asked the RAND Corporation to assess the capacity of the MHS to deliver evidence-based care for PTSD and MDD and to recommend areas in which the MHS could focus its efforts to continuously improve the quality of care provided to all service members. Specifically, this report (1) provides an overview of the PH workforce at military treatment facilities (MTFs), (2) describes the extent to which PH providers within MTFs report delivering guideline-concordant care for PTSD and MDD, (3) identifies facilitators and barriers to providing this care, and (4) provides recommendations to increase the use and monitoring of guideline-concordant care for PTSD and MDD. This report builds on previous RAND work examining the characteristics of active-component service members seen by the MHS for PTSD and MDD diagnoses and the quality of care they received using measures derived from administrative data (Hepner et al., 2016; Hepner et al., forthcoming), as well as lessons for the MHS in measuring the quality of care provided to patients with PH conditions and ensuring that this care is consistent with evidence-based clinical practice guidelines (CPGs) (Martsolf et al., 2015).

We used DoD workforce data to identify the number and mix of PH providers at MTFs. We then surveyed a representative sample of eligible providers (i.e. active-duty and government civilian) to determine the extent to which they report delivering care consistent with clinical practice guidelines for PTSD and MDD, and to identify facilitators and barriers to doing so. Semi-structured discussions with key DoD and MHS personnel provided additional context for our survey findings. Through these discussions, we collected background and perspectives on the organization of the PH workforce, approaches to monitoring demand for care and measuring performance, and quality improvement efforts for PH care.

Clinical Practice Guidelines for PTSD and MDD Care in the MHS

DoD and the U.S. Department of Veterans Affairs (VA) have been engaged in ongoing efforts to develop and promulgate guidelines to ensure that all service members receive recommended treatment for a variety of conditions commonly seen by DoD and VA health care providers. In 2009 and 2010, respectively, the VA/DoD Management of Major Depressive Disorder Working Group and the VA/DoD Management of Post-Traumatic Stress Working Group published CPGs to inform the treatment of these conditions.[1] Treatment recommendations are based on a synthesis of the research literature and expert consensus, and treatments are assigned a grade based on the strength of the evidence supporting their use. An "A" grade indicates strong evidence that an intervention improves health outcomes and that the benefits of treatment outweigh the harms. The CPGs strongly recommend that clinicians provide such interventions to eligible patients. For both PTSD and MDD, treatments in this category include specific types of psychotherapy and medication.

Strongly recommended PTSD treatments include trauma-focused cognitive behavioral therapies (i.e., prolonged exposure, cognitive processing therapy, eye movement desensitization and reprocessing), stress inoculation training, and selective serotonin reuptake inhibitors/serotonin and norepinephrine reuptake inhibitors (SSRIs/SNRIs) (Management of Post-Traumatic Stress Working Group, 2010). For MDD, strongly recommended treatments include cognitive behavioral therapy, interpersonal therapy, and problem-solving therapy, as well as certain antidepressants (Management of Major Depressive Disorder Working Group, 2009).[2]

For the purposes of our study, the VA/DoD CPG recommendations for the treatment of PTSD and MDD served as the basis for determining the extent to which MTF providers delivered high-quality, evidence-based care to service members with these conditions.

MTF PH Provider Workforce and Approaches to Treatment

Provider Mix in MTFs

The MHS relies on several types of health care providers to deliver PH care. Each service branch is responsible for its own PH workforce, assessing and monitoring PH provider performance, and the extent to which providers deliver CPG-recommended treatments. Our analyses of the PH workforce focused on psychiatrists, psychiatric nurse practitioners (PNPs), doctoral-level psychologists, and master's-level clinicians (i.e., masters-level psychologists and social workers). Other providers may deliver PH care (e.g., mental health technicians, addiction counselors). However, we focused our analysis on MTF providers most likely to deliver

---

[1]   VA/DoD CPGs include recommendations for treatment of conditions other than PTSD and MDD (e.g., acute stress disorder and dysthymia). For this report, we focused on their recommendations for PTSD and MDD only.

[2]   VA/DoD published an update to the MDD CPG as we were finalizing this report (Department of Veterans Affairs and Department of Defense, 2016); our work was guided by the 2009 practice guidelines in place at the time this research was conducted.

Table S.1
Composition of the MTF Psychological Health Provider Workforce, by Provider Type and Service Branch

Service Branch	Total Providers	Psychiatrists		PNPs		Doctoral-Level Psychologists		Master's-Level Clinicians	
		N	%	N	%	N	%	N	%
Army	2,365	320	14	89	4	638	27	1,318	56
Navy	892	193	22	67	8	354	40	278	31
Air Force	830	96	12	31	4	350	42	353	43
DoD total	4,131	612	15	189	5	1,358	33	1,972	48

NOTES: Total DoD numbers include 44 PH providers employed by the Defense Health Agency's Capital Region Medical Directorate. Master's-level clinicians include both master's-level psychologists and social workers. Data include contracted providers.

formal treatment for PTSD or MDD, as outlined in the VA/DoD CPGs, in specialty mental health care settings.

Providers may be employed in one of three ways: as an active-duty service member, as a government civilian employee, or as a civilian contractor. We collected data on the characteristics of the PH workforce from different sources, depending on the provider's employment status. We obtained data on the number and characteristics of active-duty and DoD civilian PH providers from the Defense Manpower Data Center's Health Manpower Personnel Data System. Because that system does not contain information on contractors, we requested data on contracted PH providers working in MTFs in the Army, Navy, Air Force, and Defense Health Agency.

From each source, we obtained data on provider types (e.g., psychiatrists, PNPs, psychologists, master's-level clinicians), education level (e.g., master's degree, Ph.D.), and service branch. Table S.1 shows the total number of providers in the PH MTF workforce and their representation by service branch. Note that these data include providers who deliver care at MTFs (often referred to as direct care) and do not include community providers contracted to deliver care paid for by the MHS through TRICARE (often referred to as purchased care). Master's-level clinicians, including master's-level psychologists (3 percent) and social workers (45 percent), make up the largest sector of the workforce (48 percent combined). The data revealed differences in workforce composition by service branch. For example, the Air Force has a higher proportion of doctoral-level psychologists (42 percent) than the Army (27 percent).

Most MTF PH providers are active-duty military personnel (37 percent) or civilian government employees (45 percent). Contractors constitute a relatively small portion of the overall MTF PH workforce (18 percent), but this varies by service. For example, contractors make up 38 percent of the Navy PH workforce, but only 6 percent of the Army PH workforce.

Provider Characteristics and Treatment Approaches

We conducted a survey of PH providers that assessed provider characteristics, practice characteristics, psychotherapy treatment approaches, medication management activities, training and perspectives on PTSD and MDD treatment approaches, and perceived barriers to delivering CPG-concordant care for these conditions. To achieve a final survey cohort of 500 respondents, we estimated that we needed to select a sample of approximately 1,500 PH providers.

To be eligible to participate, providers must have seen a patient with PTSD or MDD at an MTF within the previous 30 days, which we determined with an eligibility-screening item in the survey. We drew a stratified, random sample of PH providers across the MHS based on provider type, service branch, and employment status. Our survey sample included 1,489 potentially eligible PH providers who had active-duty or government civilian employment status.[3] For the purposes of our analysis, we combined psychiatrists and PNPs into a single category because there was not an adequate number of PNPs to assess this group on its own, and because both of these types of practitioners are often involved in medication management for patients with PTSD or MDD.

Providers were invited to participate and given the option to complete the survey online or by telephone. Reminder invitations were sent via regular mail and email, and invalid email addresses, telephone numbers, and mailing addresses were either updated or these providers were removed from the sample throughout the eight-week survey period, from February to April 2016. We removed respondents ineligible to participate, giving us an adjusted response rate of 39 percent (520 of 1,337 eligible providers). Because our sample and response rates by provider type were not random, we weighted the survey data to ensure that our results represented a relevant population of active-duty and government civilian PH providers.

The providers who participated in our survey had been practicing for an average of 14 years. When asked to identify their primary theoretical orientation, nearly half of master's-level clinicians and doctoral-level psychologists selected cognitive (48 percent), followed by behavioral (10 percent). Although they are separate concepts, theoretical orientation is typically directly related to the types of treatments delivered. For example, providers who endorse a cognitive or behavioral orientation may be likely to practice cognitive behavioral therapy.

Overall, providers reported seeing approximately 23 patients per week, with only a quarter of these visits occurring in a primary care setting. Among providers who had treated patients with PTSD in the previous 30 days, more than half (60 percent) reported that this group accounted for less than 25 percent of their caseload. The findings were similar for providers who had treated patients with MDD in the previous 30 days, with 62 percent reporting that these patients accounted for less than 25 percent of their caseload.

There were differences in overall caseloads, mix of patients, and care settings by service branch. For example, Army providers' caseloads had a higher proportion of patients with PTSD (45 percent) than those in the Navy (37 percent) or the Air Force (32 percent). The percentage of providers' caseloads made up of patients with MDD was not significantly different by service branch.

Delivery of Guideline-Concordant Care in the MHS

To assess delivery of guideline-concordant care, we conducted semi-structured interviews to learn about MHS approaches to monitoring the quality of care. The survey of MTF PH providers assessed self-reported use of guideline-concordant care, measurement-based care, and the facilitators and barriers to delivering guideline-concordant care.

---

[3]   Civilian contractors were not included because their participation would require Office of Management and Budget review and approval. Due to this project's time line, it was not feasible to pursue this approval.

Approaches to Monitoring Provider Performance

In an effort to standardize the assessment of PH care delivery across the MHS, in 2013, the Assistant Secretary of Defense for Health Affairs ordered the service branches to use a common system to monitor quality of care and assess provider performance. The Behavioral Health Data Portal (BHDP) is a secure, web-based system developed by the Army to collect behavioral health symptom data, patient information, diagnoses, and other visit characteristics. These data can be used to inform treatment decisions and monitor patient progress, and they can be aggregated and analyzed to, for example, identify variations in clinical outcomes or assess quality of care by PH diagnosis, treatment, provider, setting, or service branch.

In our discussions, Navy and Air Force informants noted several challenges that impeded the progress of BHDP implementation, including logistical and technical barriers, cost, a need to restructure clinics to accommodate the platform, and cultural resistance. They also cited a lack of guidance on how to implement the platform. Despite these challenges, implementation across MTFs is expected to centralize the monitoring of care quality and outcomes.

When the platform is fully implemented, BHDP data should facilitate additional efforts to understand the extent to which MTF PH providers deliver high-quality, evidence-based care to patients with PTSD and MDD consistent with VA/DoD CPG recommendations for these conditions. In the following section, we present findings from our assessment of providers' use of guideline-concordant care within MTFs in three areas: delivery of psychotherapy, medication management, and use of measurement-based care.

Provider Use of Guideline-Concordant Care
Psychotherapy Approaches for PTSD and MDD

The survey included a comprehensive list of 30 psychotherapy approaches that could be used with a PTSD patient, including the four approaches recommended in the *VA/DoD Clinical Practice Guideline for Management of Post-Traumatic Stress* (cognitive processing therapy, prolonged exposure, eye movement desensitization and reprocessing, and stress inoculation training). We created a composite of the percentage of providers who selected *any* VA/DoD-endorsed grade-A psychotherapies for PTSD as their primary approach and found that more than half of providers (59 percent) selected at least one.[4]

We found significant differences in the delivery of CPG-concordant care for PTSD by provider type and service branch. Doctoral-level psychologists (78 percent) were more likely than master's-level clinicians (56 percent) and psychiatrists/PNPs (21 percent) to select a treatment identified as effective for PTSD in the VA/DoD CPG for posttraumatic stress as their primary psychotherapy approach. Air Force providers (80 percent) were significantly more likely than Army (55 percent) and Navy (54 percent) providers to select a primary approach for PTSD psychotherapy that was a grade-A treatment.

Our survey also included a comprehensive list of 30 psychotherapy approaches that could be used with an MDD patient, including the three approaches recommended in the VA/DoD CPG as first-line psychotherapies for uncomplicated MDD (cognitive behavioral therapy,

---

[4] Although the survey included cognitive behavioral therapy, we excluded this approach from our analysis because we could not be certain whether it was trauma-focused, as recommended by the VA/DoD CPG. This number would increase to 79 percent if providers indicated *trauma-focused* cognitive behavioral therapy, specifically, as their primary psychotherapy approach for patients with PTSD.

interpersonal therapy, and problem-solving therapy).[5] We created a composite of the percentage of providers who selected *any* VA/DoD-endorsed psychotherapies as their primary MDD psychotherapy approach and found that 61 percent selected at least one. We found significant differences in the delivery of CPG-concordant care by provider type but not by service branch. Specifically, master's-level clinicians (67 percent) and doctoral-level psychologists (62 percent) had a similar likelihood of selecting a strongly recommended psychotherapy for MDD as their primary approach, and both these groups were more likely to do so than psychiatrists/PNPs (45.3 percent).

Because self-reported primary therapy approaches may be vulnerable to socially desirable responding, we asked about the specific techniques that had been used with a patient as a means of indirectly assessing whether a guideline-concordant psychotherapy had been delivered. We hypothesized that this approach would be less influenced by social desirability. We expected that a smaller proportion of providers would report delivering all core elements of guideline-concordant psychotherapies than would indicate that a given psychotherapy was their primary approach. In fact, we found the opposite. For example, twice as many providers indicated that they had delivered all core cognitive processing therapy techniques than claimed that cognitive processing therapy was their primary psychotherapy approach, and 96 percent of providers indicated that they had delivered all interpersonal therapy techniques even though use of interpersonal therapy as a primary approach was quite rare (< 1 percent). It may be that the items designed to measure the core techniques of specific therapies instead captured relatively common therapy techniques that are shared across therapies. This suggests that additional scale development work is required.

Medication Management for PTSD and MDD

We asked survey respondents to provide details on medications currently prescribed to patients with PTSD or MDD they had seen in the previous 30 days. These items addressed the types and number of psychopharmacological medications prescribed to patients with these conditions. The VA/DoD CPG recommendations for treatment of PTSD strongly recommends SSRIs and SNRIs as grade-A medications for eligible patients; it also lists medications with "at least fair levels of effectiveness" (grade B) and medications it deems ineffective or potentially harmful to patients with PTSD (grade D). Nearly 90 percent of providers who had prescribed medication indicated they had currently prescribed a grade-A medication to their most recent PTSD patient, but a clinically significant minority (11 percent) reported currently prescribing a medication that CPG guidelines recommend against—specifically, medications with the potential to cause harm or worsen PTSD outcomes.

The VA/DoD CPG for MDD strongly recommends SSRIs, SNRIs, bupropion, and mirtazapine as grade-A medications for eligible patients with MDD; it also lists grade-B medications with limited evidence of effectiveness. Overall, 97 percent of prescribers reported that their most recent MDD patient was currently prescribed at least one grade-A medication, and only 1 percent were currently prescribed a grade-B medication. Providers also indicated that 69 percent of MDD patients were currently prescribed more than one medication, with

---

[5]   Our analyses focused on these three approaches. The CPG identifies two other grade-A psychotherapies for MDD but limits the recommendation for their use to a specific subgroup of patients: behavioral therapy/behavioral activation for inpatients and patients with severe depression and electroconvulsive therapy for a highly specific subset of patients with severe MDD (e.g., catatonia or other psychotic symptoms).

12 percent currently prescribed four or more. As the number of prescriptions goes up, the probability that any one of them is classified as a grade-A medication will also rise. This may partially explain the high reported rates of grade-A medication use.

Provider Use of Measurement-Based Care

Screening and monitoring patient symptoms with validated instruments—another contributor to high-quality care—can inform treatment planning and subsequent adjustments. The majority of surveyed providers reported that either they or their support staff "always" screened new patients for PTSD (71 percent) and MDD (79 percent) with a validated screening instrument. Army providers were significantly more likely than Air Force providers to screen new patients for PTSD with a validated screening instrument. However, this pattern was reversed for MDD, with Air Force providers more likely than both Army and Navy providers to screen for MDD with a validated instrument. Overall, fewer providers (58 percent) reported using a validated instrument on patient symptoms to inform treatment plan adjustments. These results suggest that most providers may be routinely screening these patients, but fewer use validated instruments to monitor treatment outcomes.

Facilitators and Barriers to Providing Guideline-Concordant Care

Our survey and key informant discussions elicited information on perceived facilitators and barriers to providing care that was consistent with VA/DoD CPG recommendations for treating PTSD and MDD. Both providers and key informants indicated that training and supervision in evidence-based interventions was a potential facilitator, but a lack of such training could be a barrier. According to our key informants, the Army and Air Force have established training initiatives, but there appears to be no such program in the Navy.

Our survey results indicated that, among respondents who delivered any psychotherapy in the previous 30 days, the majority had received minimally adequate training/supervision in at least one grade-A PTSD psychotherapy (77 percent) or MDD psychotherapy (69 percent).[6] We also inquired about providers' level of confidence in delivering evidence-based treatments and found that they were most confident in their ability to prescribe medication for PTSD (94 percent) and MDD (96 percent). However, confidence levels were lower for the CPG-endorsed psychotherapies for each of these conditions.

Key informants pointed to patient-level factors as barriers to providing high-quality PH care, such as patients' ability to balance appointment and treatment schedules with their military duties. Providers' caseloads may also limit the frequency with which providers can see patients. However, more than 80 percent of survey respondents reported seeing patients for eight or more sessions, suggesting that most patients are receiving at least the minimum number of psychotherapy sessions recommended for PTSD or MDD. Finally, our key informants cited a lack of information sharing among providers and locations as a barrier to high-quality care, though DoD is taking steps to mitigate these challenges.

To better gauge providers' perspectives, our survey contained 26 items that assessed potential barriers to delivering guideline-concordant care for PTSD and MDD. Table S.2 shows the top six perceived barriers to providing guideline-concordant care as cited by survey participants. Barriers to training were the top two barriers. Specifically, providers reported that

---

[6] To identify the proportion of providers who may have this capacity, we defined *minimally adequate training/supervision* as more than eight hours of training and at least one hour of supervision in a given modality.

Table S.2
Top Barriers to Delivery of Guideline-Concordant Care for PTSD and MDD

Response	Percentage of Providers Who Strongly Agree/Strongly Disagree[a]
Limitations on travel prevent me from receiving additional training.	31.7
I have protected time in my schedule to attend workshops/seminars to improve my clinical skills. (reverse-scored)	28.6
Nonspecific aspects of therapy, like good rapport, are the best predictors of treatment success.	25.7
I don't have the time in my schedule to see patients as often as I would like.	24.7
My patients' military duties limit their ability to receive appropriate care (e.g., patient PCS, deployment, irregular work schedules).	17.6
I am well-supported by case managers (e.g., coordinating interdisciplinary care, follow-up with patients who do not attend appointments). (reverse-scored)	17.4

NOTES: N = 503. Due to missing values, the number of responses for each item ranged from 498 to 503. PCS = permanent change of station.

[a] Some items were reverse-scored.

limits on travel and the lack of protected time affected their ability to access additional professional training.

Delivering Guideline-Concordant Care for PTSD and MDD in MTFs: Key Findings

Our analysis of MTF workforce data, responses to our provider survey, and discussions with key informants yielded a number of findings that highlight focus areas for future improvement efforts.

Most Providers Reported Using Guideline-Concordant Psychotherapies, but Use Varied by Provider Type

Overall, 59 percent of psychotherapy providers identified a guideline-concordant psychotherapy as their primary approach for treatment for patients with PTSD. Psychologists (78 percent) were more likely than master's-level clinicians (56 percent) and psychiatrists/PNPs (21 percent) to select a guideline-concordant psychotherapy as their primary approach of treatment for patients with PTSD. With the available data, we were able to only partially explain this gap between provider types, and this could be an area for future research. Although not all providers indicated that their primary PTSD psychotherapy approach was CPG-concordant, there nonetheless appeared to be a depth of familiarity with these approaches among master's-level clinicians and psychologists, 85 to 91 percent of whom had delivered a CPG-concordant psychotherapy in the past.

These patterns were similar for the treatment of MDD, with more psychologists (62 percent) and master's-level clinicians (67 percent) than psychiatrists/PNPs (45 percent) selecting a guideline-concordant psychotherapy as their primary psychotherapy approach. However, a substantial majority of providers (79–94 percent) had delivered a guideline-concordant therapy for MDD in the past, suggesting that a lack of familiarity with these treatments may not be a primary barrier to delivering high-quality care for MDD.

Nearly All Psychiatrists and PNPs Reported Using Guideline-Concordant Medications to Treat PTSD and MDD, but Most Patients Received Multiple Psychopharmacologic Medications

Nearly 90 percent of psychiatrists/PNPs who had written prescriptions for their most recent PTSD patients prescribed at least one grade-A medication; this was true for 97 percent of those who treated MDD patients. However, providers reported that 84 percent of PTSD patients had been prescribed more than one psychopharmacological medication, and nearly a quarter had been prescribed four or more medications. Among all PTSD patients prescribed medication, 11 percent were receiving medications indicated as harmful to treatment progress according to VA/DoD CPG recommendations for PTSD (grade D). Providers also indicated that 69 percent of MDD patients received more than one medication, with 12 percent receiving four or more. Additional research is needed to determine whether these patterns of prescribing are appropriate.

Most Providers Reported Routinely Screening Patients for PTSD and MDD, but Fewer Used Validated Instruments to Monitor Treatment Outcomes

The majority of providers reported that they always screened for PTSD (71 percent) and MDD (79 percent) with a validated screening instrument, but fewer providers (58 percent) reported using a validated instrument to monitor patient symptoms and inform adjustments to treatment plans, with differences by service branch. More work is needed to identify the potential benefits of increasing the use of these tools and reasons for the variability in their use.

The Majority of Therapists Reported Receiving at Least Minimal Training/Supervision in a Guideline-Concordant Psychotherapy, but Some Reported Difficulty Accessing Additional Training

The majority of therapists received minimally adequate training and supervision in at least one CPG-concordant psychotherapy for PTSD (77 percent) and MDD (69 percent). However, it is important to note that we applied a lenient definition of minimal adequacy (at least eight hours of training and at least one hour of supervision). We also found differences in providers' confidence in their ability to deliver various types of therapies. Additional training could increase providers' confidence and may, in turn, increase delivery of these recommended treatments.

Some Providers Reported Seeing Patients Infrequently

On average, MTF providers reported seeing 23 patients per week. However, some providers indicated that their caseloads precluded them from seeing their patients as often as they would like. Most psychotherapies are tested across a given number of weekly sessions, and it remains unclear whether patients seen for psychotherapy visits less frequently than weekly receive the full benefit of these treatments. A sensitivity analysis revealed that among psychotherapy-only providers, 45 and 49 percent saw their PTSD and MDD patients weekly (respectively), with the remaining providers seeing patients less often. Further, among providers who delivered only medication management, the modal frequency was monthly (44 and 39 percent for PTSD and MDD patients, respectively). Additionally, a fifth of providers reported seeing patients for fewer than eight sessions. This may not be adequate for patients to benefit from the treatment provided.

Key Strengths and Limitations

This study has a number of key strengths, notably that a comprehensive provider survey was fielded across service branches and several types of PH providers who deliver care for PTSD or MDD in MTFs. However, some limitations should be noted. The provider survey did not include contracted civilian personnel or purchased care providers. Survey sampling relied on existing provider data, which could have resulted in inappropriate exclusion or inclusion of providers. The survey relied on providers' self-report of their approach and perspectives on treating patients with PTSD or MDD, which may have been subject to bias (e.g., social desirability or recall bias). As a result, responses to survey items may not directly correspond with actual provider practice. Finally, while key informant discussions provided important context for interpreting survey results, the limited number of key informant discussions did not fully capture the state of PH care. Despite these limitations, this report provides a comprehensive assessment of providers' perspectives on their capacity to deliver PH care within MTFs and presents detailed results by provider type and service branch.

Recommendations to Guide Improvements in PH Care Across the MHS

Overall, MTF providers are delivering high-quality, CPG-concordant care to patients with PTSD and MDD, but gaps and barriers remain. Our findings pointed to four primary recommendations to guide improvements in care for PTSD, MDD, and other PH conditions within the MHS and to ensure that the care provided is consistent with VA/DoD guidelines.

Recommendation 1. Maximize the Effectiveness of Psychotherapy Training and Reduce Barriers

Recommendation 1a. Adopt a Systematic, Broad-Based Approach to Training and Certification in Guideline-Concordant Therapies, and Track Provider Progress

As the MHS and service branches continue efforts to increase implementation of guideline-concordant psychotherapy, it may be useful to adopt a systematic approach. While key informants described multiple training efforts, it appears there is no formal tracking system or provider certification process MHS-wide or by service branch to ensure that MTFs have the appropriate mix of provider competence to ensure availability of guideline-concordant psychotherapies. Certification in a particular type of psychotherapy indicates that a provider has received training and clinical supervision and ultimately demonstrated competence in delivering that psychotherapy. This process is separate from the traditional credentialing process that ensures a provider has the appropriate degree and license. Tracking provider certifications that indicate competence would allow training efforts to be targeted to particular providers or address a need for a particular type of psychotherapy. It could also guide ongoing quality improvement. Identifying and addressing provider-specific barriers to use of guideline-concordant therapies will be key strategies in improving quality of PH care.

Recommendation 1b. Reduce Barriers to Receiving Training in Guideline-Concordant Therapies

Among the multiple potential barriers to providing guideline-concordant treatment assessed in the provider survey, obstacles to training were the top two barriers, including limits on travel and lack of protected time for trainings. The MHS and service branch leadership should consider one or more of the following policy changes to increase access to trainings and reduce barriers to attending these trainings. First, travel restrictions for training could be lifted or reduced. Second, the MHS could increase delivery of onsite trainings that do not require travel. Finally, the MHS could increase the use of web-based trainings. While these strategies would increase training opportunities, they may not address the second major training barrier identified, which is lack of protected time to participate in trainings. Providers may need additional support from their leadership to allow this protected time. This could be a challenge if provider incentives focus on number of patient visits rather than enhancing skills. Allowing for time to receive supervision/consultation following didactic training will help to ensure providers achieve competence in delivering the therapy.

Recommendation 2. Monitor the Frequency and Duration of Psychotherapy Treatment

Our results raised questions about whether PH providers are able to see patients with PTSD or MDD with the frequency and duration that may be associated with improved outcomes. These results highlight the importance of understanding these patterns to ensure access and availability to psychotherapy appointments. This finding, along with findings from a separate study in which MHS patients reported (Tanielian et al., 2016) frustration over not being able to get timely follow-up appointments, suggests that specific efforts to address the timeliness and frequency of psychotherapy visits is warranted. Toward that end, the MHS should routinely monitor frequency and duration of psychotherapy treatment. This is consistent with recommendations from a recent RAND report that the MHS can improve at providing an adequate amount of treatment for service members beginning a new treatment episode for PTSD or depression. This report included data applying a quality measure that assessed whether service members received at least four psychotherapy visits or two medication management visits in the first eight weeks of beginning their treatment. A modified version of this measure could track frequency and duration of psychotherapy visits. Monitoring this measure would increase emphasis on timely ongoing appointments and balance existing incentives that focus on timely first appointments. While the optimum number and timing of visits is not certain, particularly for an individual patient, observing variation across providers, MTFs, and service branches and investigating the causes of these variations could guide quality improvement. Further, it would allow the MHS to gain a better understanding of the role that patient schedules, preferences, and response to treatment play in attenuating or increasing frequency and duration of treatment. Understanding "no shows" and cancellation rates may lead to implementation of proactive strategies to reduce these rates (e.g., reminder calls, no show policies). To the extent that the data reveal that capacity constraints are driving the inability to meet frequency and duration expectations, MHS leaders will need to consider options for expanding capacity and access (Tanielian et al., 2016).

Recommendation 3. Expand Monitoring of Treatment Outcomes and Use That Information to Improve Quality of Care for PH Conditions

Outcome monitoring across MTFs using BHDP is a promising effort that could be a core tool to monitor and improve outcomes. Providers reported using validated measures more frequently for screening than for informing adjustments to treatment. As the MHS works to increase monitoring of symptoms for patients with PH conditions, it will be important that providers understand how to use this information to inform treatment planning and adjustments to treatment. Providers may need additional training and feedback about how to use the information generated from BHDP at the patient level. Alternatively, real time Clinical Decision Support tools and other technologies can help guide clinical decisionmaking and engage patients. Further, additional training and feedback could be used to ensure providers evaluate their own practice. Encouraging providers to consider their own treatment outcomes, along with ways to improve (e.g., taking advantages of training opportunities), could engage providers in quality improvement. In addition, the MHS can expand use of BHDP data to guide quality improvement efforts. These data could identify PH providers and MTFs that are "outliers" in terms of their ability to obtain improved outcomes (both higher performers and possible lower performers). These data could be linked with process quality measures that would indicate whether the care the provider delivers is typically guideline-concordant and consider whether care could be improved.

Recommendation 4. Develop a Systematic, MHS-Wide Approach to Increasing the Delivery of Guideline-Concordant PH Care Through a Continuous Quality Improvement Strategy

Because service branches have the responsibility for care delivery, staffing, and training providers, there are few MHS-wide efforts to systematically monitor and improve PH care. BHDP is a notable exception and will provide visibility across the MHS on important aspects of the delivery of guideline-concordant care, including symptom monitoring and utilization. The key to increasing the capacity of the MHS to deliver such care, however, is developing and implementing system-wide continuous quality improvement efforts. While we are aware of several service branch–specific efforts, implementing MHS-wide efforts may increase efficiency and shared learning across the service branches.

Monitoring the quality of care is a critical step in ensuring that all patients receive high-quality care. However, using the data effectively and systematically to implement quality improvement initiatives is equally important. By continuously gathering and using data at the system level, as recommended above, the MHS will be able to identify areas for improvement, develop and test strategies for improvement, and then implement those strategies across services. To effectively implement systemic quality improvement efforts across the MHS, service branches and the Defense Health Agency (DHA) will need to determine how to allocate responsibility for these efforts and to assure that those accountable for quality at each level (from MTF to service branch) receive appropriate training in quality improvement tools and procedures. While DHA is collecting data and monitoring quality across service branches, past efforts to improve care have occurred within service branches, rather than across the MHS as a whole. We recommend that MHS policymakers consider mechanisms for system-wide improvements, which should increase efficiency and reduce variability in the delivery of care.

This study expanded on previous RAND work on quality of care for PH conditions by describing the PH workforce at MTFs, examining the extent to which MTF providers report care for PTSD and MDD is consistent with clinical practice guidelines, and identifying facilitators and barriers to providing this care. These findings highlight areas of strength for the MHS, as well as areas that should be targeted for quality improvement. The results presented here can inform how the MHS and service branches can support continuous improvement in the PH care the MHS delivers.

Acknowledgments

We gratefully acknowledge the support of our project sponsors, CDR Angela Williams and Kate McGraw, and staff at DCoE. We also acknowledge those who provided feedback on drafts of our survey instrument, including Charles Engel, LTC JoEllen Fielden, Charles Hoge, Lisa Jaycox, Lisa Meredith, and David Riggs. We thank the staff at Davis Research for their assistance fielding the provider survey, particularly Jason Kerns, who oversaw that effort. We appreciate the valuable insights we received from Mary Jo Larson and Lisa Meredith. We addressed their constructive critiques as part of RAND's rigorous quality assurance process to improve the quality of this report. We also thank Lauren Skrabala, Laura Pavlock-Albright, and Tiffany Hruby for their assistance in preparing this report, and Terry Marsh for overseeing human-subjects and regulatory protocols and approvals for the project. Finally, we extend our gratitude to the many DoD officials who participated in our key informant discussions and shared information about their experiences, along with the more than 500 psychological health providers who participated in our survey.

Abbreviations

BH	behavioral health
BHDP	Behavioral Health Data Portal
CBT	cognitive behavioral therapy
CPG	clinical practice guideline
CPT	cognitive processing therapy
DCoE	Defense Centers of Excellence for Psychological Health and Traumatic Brain Injury
DHA	Defense Health Agency
DoD	U.S. Department of Defense
EMDR	eye movement desensitization and reprocessing
HA	Health Affairs
HMPDS	Health Manpower Personnel Data System
IPT	interpersonal psychotherapy
MDD	major depressive disorder
MHS	Military Health System
MTF	military treatment facility
OASD/HA	Office of the Assistant Secretary of Defense for Health Affairs
OMB	Office of Management and Budget
PCS	permanent change of station
PE	prolonged exposure
PH	psychological health
PNP	psychiatric nurse practitioner
PTSD	posttraumatic stress disorder

SE   standard error

SNRI   serotonin and norepinephrine reuptake inhibitor

SSRI   selective serotonin reuptake inhibitor

VA   U.S. Department of Veterans Affairs

CHAPTER ONE

Introduction

Providing high-quality treatment and improving outcomes for individuals with psychological health (PH) problems are high-priority goals for the Military Health System (MHS) (Obama, 2012). As psychological health is vital to force readiness, the U.S. Department of Defense (DoD) has made a concerted effort to prevent and treat PH conditions among service members (Department of Defense, Department of Veterans Affairs, Department of Health and Human Services, 2013). Since 2001, more than 2.6 million U.S. military personnel have been deployed to support Operation Enduring Freedom, Operation Iraqi Freedom, and Operation New Dawn (Institute of Medicine, 2014). The estimated rate of PH diagnoses among active-duty service members has increased 65 percent since the beginning of these conflicts (Blakeley and Jansen, 2013). To meet the increased demand for PH care, the MHS has increased the size of its PH workforce (U.S. Government Accountability Office, 2015), established training programs in evidence-based treatments (Borah et al., 2013; Center for Deployment Psychology, undated), developed innovative programs addressing PH needs (Weinick et al., 2011), and implemented other approaches to enhance the availability and quality of PH care. Whether these efforts have resulted in a system of care that meets the needs of service members with PH conditions is unclear, and little is known about the facilitators and barriers affecting the ability of the MHS to deliver high-quality, evidence-based PH care.

To address these questions, the DoD's Defense Centers of Excellence for Psychological Health and Traumatic Brain Injury (DCoE) asked the RAND Corporation to assess the capacity of the MHS to deliver high-quality care for posttraumatic stress disorder (PTSD) and major depressive disorder (MDD), two of the most common PH conditions diagnosed and treated in the MHS. *This report (1) provides an overview of the PH workforce at military treatment facilities (MTFs), (2) examines the extent to which care for PTSD and MDD in the MTFs is consistent with clinical practice guidelines (CPGs), and (3) identifies facilitators and barriers to providing this care.* Understanding workforce capacity, particularly from the provider perspective, is an important step toward ensuring the success of future improvement efforts, including the development of ongoing processes to monitor and increase the availability of high-quality PH care.

In this introductory chapter, we provide an overview of the prevalence of PTSD and MDD in the MHS, describe recommended treatments, and provide a rationale for assessing and monitoring capacity to provide high-quality care for these conditions.

Providing Effective Care for PTSD and MDD for Service Members

The burden of PH conditions among service members in the U.S. military remains a pressing issue. Estimates of PTSD prevalence rates in U.S. military populations range from 5 to 24.5 percent. Research indicates that rates are higher for service members who deployed to Iraq in support of Operation Iraqi Freedom than for those who deployed to Afghanistan in support of Operation Enduring Freedom, higher among women than among men in the military, and higher for individual service members after deployment relative to before (Fulton et al., 2015; Hoge, Auchterlonie, and Milliken, 2006; Hoge et al., 2004; Maguen et al., 2010; Milliken, Auchterlonie, and Hoge, 2007; Ramchand et al., 2008; Ramchand et al., 2010; Ramchand et al., 2015; Schell and Marshall, 2008; Smith et al., 2007; Wells et al., 2011). Prevalence estimates for depression among service members range from 7.9 to 15 percent, with higher rates reported after deployment, among women relative to men, and among reserve service members relative to those in the active component (Hoge, Auchterlonie, and Milliken, 2006; Hoge et al., 2004; Maguen et al., 2010; Milliken, Auchterlonie, and Hoge, 2007; Ramchand et al., 2008; Ramchand et al., 2015; Schell and Marshall, 2008). These numbers represent a substantial need for care.

Effective treatments for PTSD and MDD exist, and DoD and the U.S. Department of Veterans Affairs (VA) have been engaged in ongoing efforts to develop and promulgate CPGs to ensure that all service members receive recommended treatment. In 2009 and 2010, respectively, the VA/DoD Management of Major Depressive Disorder Working Group and the VA/DoD Management of Post-Traumatic Stress Working Group published CPGs to inform the treatment of DoD and VA beneficiaries with those conditions.[1] In the following sections, we provide a brief overview of these guidelines and efforts to estimate whether service members receive guideline-concordant care.

Clinical Practice Guidelines for PTSD and MDD

VA/DoD CPGs provide treatment recommendations based on a synthesis of research literature and expert consensus.[2] Treatment recommendations are assigned grades according to the strength of the evidence (Table 1.1). An "A" grade is a strong recommendation for clinicians to provide the intervention to eligible patients, meaning there is strong evidence that the intervention improves health outcomes and that the benefits of treatment outweigh the harms. For both PTSD and MDD, the guidelines strongly recommend treatment involving specific types of psychotherapy or medication (Table 1.2). Throughout this report, we use the descriptions *grade A* and *strongly recommended* interchangeably.

Strongly Recommended Treatments for PTSD

Strongly recommended psychotherapies for PTSD include trauma-focused cognitive behavioral therapies and stress inoculation training (Management of Post-Traumatic Stress Working Group, 2010). Trauma-focused cognitive behavioral therapies use cognitive and/or behavioral techniques to alleviate PTSD symptoms. Specific techniques include exposure, which

---

[1]   DoD/VA CPGs include recommendations for treatment of conditions other than PTSD and MDD (e.g., acute stress disorder and dysthymia). For this report, we focused on their recommendations for PTSD and MDD only.

[2]   DoD/VA CPGs note that treatment recommendations reflect the best available information to guide provider decision-making, but they are not intended to define a standard of care, as variations in practice can occur based on several factors.

Table 1.1
Strength of Evidence Grades

Strength of Recommendation	Definition
A	A strong recommendation that clinicians provide the intervention to eligible patients. Good evidence was found that the intervention improves important health outcomes and concludes that benefits substantially outweigh harm.
B	A recommendation that clinicians provide (the service) to eligible patients.
C	No recommendation for or against the routine provision of the intervention is made. At least fair evidence was found that the intervention can improve health outcomes but concludes that the balance of benefits and harms is too close to justify a general recommendation.
D	Recommendation is made against routinely providing the intervention to asymptomatic patients. At least fair evidence was found that the intervention is ineffective or that the harms outweigh benefits.
I	The conclusion is that the evidence is insufficient to recommend for or against routinely providing the intervention. Evidence that the intervention is effective is lacking, of poor quality, or conflicting, and the balance of benefits and harms cannot be determined.

SOURCE: Management of Post-Traumatic Stress Working Group, 2010, p. 7.

Table 1.2
VA/DoD Strongly Recommended Treatments for PTSD and MDD

Condition	Psychotherapy	Pharmacotherapy
PTSD	Trauma-focused cognitive behavioral therapies (i.e., prolonged exposure, cognitive processing therapy, eye movement desensitization and reprocessing), stress inoculation training	Selective serotonin reuptake inhibitors (SSRIs), serotonin-norepinephrine reuptake inhibitors (SNRIs)
MDD	First-line psychotherapy for uncomplicated MDD: cognitive behavioral therapy, interpersonal therapy, problem-solving therapy	SSRIs (except fluvoxamine), SNRIs, bupropion, mirtazapine
	Other psychotherapy: behavior therapy/behavioral activation for patients with severe depression, electroconvulsive therapy for a highly specific subset of patients with severe MDD (e.g., catatonia or other psychotic symptoms)	

SOURCE: Management of Post-Traumatic Stress Working Group, 2010; Management of Major Depressive Disorder Working Group, 2009.

reduces anxiety by acclimating patients to trauma reminders; cognitive restructuring, during which patients discuss thoughts related to the traumatic event and adjust cognitive distortions; anxiety management techniques such as relaxation training; emotional regulation; and distress tolerance (Management of Post-Traumatic Stress Working Group, 2010). Between-session practice assignments (often called homework) are an important component of these therapies. Cognitive processing therapy, prolonged exposure, and eye movement desensitization and reprocessing are grade-A treatment modalities under the umbrella of trauma-focused cognitive behavioral therapy. Stress inoculation training is a general anxiety-management therapy that includes such techniques as assertiveness training, positive thinking, and thought stopping. Although stress inoculation training incorporates some cognitive behavioral therapy techniques, this modality is generally not trauma-focused (Management of Post-Traumatic Stress Working Group, 2010). The American Psychiatric Association also endorses cognitive behavioral therapy as an effective treatment for PTSD symptoms (American Psychiatric Association, 2004).

The VA/DoD CPG for post-traumatic stress also grades the strength of the evidence for specific PTSD pharmacotherapies (Management of Post-Traumatic Stress Working Group, 2010). Evidence from numerous randomized control trials and meta-analyses of those trials supports the use of SSRIs and SNRIs in treating PTSD (Brady et al., 2000; Davidson et al., 2001; Foa, Davidson, and Frances, 1999; Jonas et al., 2013; Stein, Ipser, and Seedat, 2009). As such, the VA/DoD CPG assigns an A grade to SSRIs/SNRIs for PTSD treatment, indicating that these treatment options are strongly recommended (Management of Post-Traumatic Stress Working Group, 2010). The American Psychiatric Association and the International Society for Traumatic Stress Studies concur that SSRIs/SNRIs are effective treatment options for PTSD (American Psychiatric Association, 2004; Benedek et al., 2009; Foa, Davidson, and Frances, 1999).

Strongly Recommended Treatments for MDD

For MDD, the VA/DoD CPG considers cognitive behavioral therapy, interpersonal therapy, and problem-solving therapy as grade-A psychotherapy treatment options and recommends them as first-line psychotherapies, specifically for the treatment of uncomplicated major depression (Management of Major Depressive Disorder Working Group, 2009). Cognitive behavioral therapy emphasizes behavioral change and cognitive restructuring by encouraging patients to question negative thoughts and uncover the root cause of maladaptive thinking (Management of Major Depressive Disorder Working Group, 2009). Cognitive behavioral therapy sessions are highly structured and instruction-focused; therapists also assign between-session homework assignments for patients to practice newly acquired skills (Management of Major Depressive Disorder Working Group, 2009). Interpersonal therapy focuses on resolving relational conflicts and improving role-functioning to reduce depressive symptoms (American Psychiatric Association, 2010). Interpersonal therapy centers on four major domains: interpersonal loss, role conflict, role change, and interpersonal skills (Management of Major Depressive Disorder Working Group, 2009). Problem-solving therapy is a short-term intervention strongly recommended by the VA/DoD CPG for those with mild to moderate MDD. Particularly useful in primary care settings, this treatment involves the clinician and patient collaborating to identify key problem areas and develop appropriate coping tools (Management of Major Depressive Disorder Working Group, 2009). Clinical guidelines from the American Psychiatric Association support cognitive behavioral therapy and interpersonal therapy as effective psychotherapy treatments for MDD (Management of Major Depressive Disorder Working Group, 2009), while the Institute for Clinical Improvement Systems endorses cognitive behavioral therapy, interpersonal therapy, and problem-solving therapy (Trangle et al., 2016).

The VA/DoD CPG for MDD strongly recommends antidepressants as a pharmacotherapy treatment option. Recommended antidepressants include SSRIs, SNRIs, bupropion, and mirtazapine (Management of Major Depressive Disorder Working Group, 2009). This recommendation is in accordance with guidelines from the American Psychiatric Association and the Institute for Clinical Systems Improvement, both of which endorse antidepressants as an effective pharmacotherapy treatment for MDD (American Psychiatric Association, 2010; Trangle et al., 2016). VA/DoD published an update to the MDD CPG as we were finalizing this report (Department of Veterans Affairs and Department of Defense, 2016); our work was guided by the 2009 practice guidelines in place at the time this research was conducted.

Delivering Guideline-Concordant Care for PTSD and MDD in the MHS

Recent analyses show variation in the quality of care that the MHS provides for PTSD and MDD (Hepner et al., 2016; U.S. Government Accountability Office, 2016). For example, one recent study used quality measures, also called performance measures, to assess how well health care is being delivered in the MHS. These quality measures are applied by operationalizing aspects of care recommended by CPGs using administrative data, medical records, clinical registries, patient or clinician surveys, and other data sources. The study found that the MHS outperformed other health care systems on quality measures assessing whether patients with PTSD or MDD who had been discharged from a psychiatric hospitalization received timely outpatient follow-up (Hepner et al., 2016). However, it found that the MHS could increase the amount of treatment (either psychotherapy or medication management visits) provided to service members who are beginning a new treatment episode for PTSD or depression. Similarly, fewer than half of service members received a follow-up visit within 30 days of starting new medication treatment for PTSD or depression (Hepner et al., 2016). Recent analyses have also suggested that fewer than half of service members who received psychotherapy had documentation in their medical record indicating that these were guideline-concordant, evidence-based treatments (45 percent for PTSD; 30 percent for depression; Hepner et al., 2017).

In a report on the quality of care provided to military personnel, the Institute of Medicine noted wide variation in PTSD care across service branches (Institute of Medicine, 2014), highlighting that PTSD management within DoD "appear[ed] to be local, ad hoc, incremental and crisis-driven with little planning devoted to the development of a long-range, population approach for the disorder."

While these reports provide valuable information about gaps in PH care in the MHS, they do not identify why these inadequacies occur. A clear understanding of the factors that either support or create barriers to high-quality care is critical for developing effective, feasible solutions that address disparities in care.

Research Objectives

A core component of the capacity of the MHS to provide guideline-concordant care for PTSD and MDD is the extent to which PH providers working in MTFs are currently providing such care, whether they have received adequate training in recommended treatments, and what barriers they encounter to providing high-quality care. Toward this end, this report

1. **Describes the PH workforce at MTFs.** We used DoD workforce data to provide an overview of the number and mix of PH providers in each of the service branches, with a focus on psychiatrists, psychiatric nurse practitioners (PNPs), Ph.D.-level psychologists, and master's-level clinicians.
2. **Describes the extent to which PH providers within MTFs report delivering guideline-concordant care for PTSD and MDD.** We surveyed a representative sample of eligible MTF PH providers (i.e., psychiatrists, PNPs, psychologists, social workers, and other master's-level clinicians who were active duty or government civilians). Civilian contractors were not included, due to the additional regulatory requirements that were not feasible to complete during the project time line. The survey assessed the extent to which providers reported using guideline-concordant practices to treat adults

with PTSD or MDD. To provide context for these results, we also conducted semi-structured discussions with key personnel across DoD and the MHS.

3. **Identifies facilitators and barriers to providing guideline-concordant care for PTSD and MDD.** The PH provider survey and semi-structured discussions with key personnel allowed us to identify factors that support providers in using guideline-concordant practices, barriers that interfere with providing this care, and targets for quality-improvement efforts.

4. **Develops recommendations to increase the use and monitoring of guideline-concordant care for PTSD and MDD.** Based on our findings, we developed targeted recommendations to support efforts to improve outcomes for service members and other adult beneficiaries with these conditions.

While this report includes important information about the PH provider workforce delivering care in MTFs, this report does not provide a complete description of all aspects of PH care organization and delivery in the MHS and service branches. The principal methods described in this report were developed and prioritized in consultation with DCoE, the sponsor of this work. Further, this report does not include contractors delivering care at MTFs, or purchased care providers delivering care in the community paid for by the MHS through TRICARE. Finally, this report focuses on the delivery of recommended treatments to adult patients diagnosed with PTSD or MDD and does not address screening and assessment for these conditions.

Organization of This Report

This report provides an assessment of the composition of the MTF PH workforce and its capacity to deliver evidence-based care for PTSD and MDD. The remainder of the report is organized as follows. Chapter Two details the methods and data sources used for analysis. Chapter Three describes the organization and delivery of PH care within MTFs and the size and characteristics of this PH workforce. Chapter Four highlights efforts to monitor the delivery of guideline-concordant care and presents findings on the extent to which such care is provided for PTSD and MDD within MTFs. Chapter Five describes facilitators and barriers to delivering guideline-concordant care for these PH conditions. Chapter Six presents our conclusions and recommendations. Three appendixes include additional technical details on our survey sampling and weighting approaches (Appendix A), the domains and measures included in the provider survey (Appendix B), the complete fielded survey (Appendix C), and the guide for our semi-structured discussions with key informants (Appendix D).

CHAPTER TWO

Methods

In this chapter, we describe the methods used to build a profile of the PH workforce at MTFs, assess the extent to which MTF PH providers reported delivering CPG-concordant care for PTSD and MDD, and identify facilitators and barriers to providing this care. We also describe our use of key informant discussions to contextualize survey results within current MHS approaches to promoting and monitoring the quality of PH care. All study methods were approved by RAND's Human Subjects Protection Committee, as well as by the U.S. Army Medical Research and Materiel Command's Human Research Protection Office. In addition, the PH provider survey was licensed by Washington Headquarters Services (DD-USA[OT]2594) as an approved DoD internal information collection procedure.

Provider Data

The MHS relies on several different types of health care providers to deliver PH care. Our analyses of the MTF PH workforce focused on psychiatrists, PNPs, psychologists, social workers, and other master's-level clinicians. While other providers may deliver PH care (e.g., mental health technicians, addiction counselors), we focused on providers who were most likely to deliver formal treatment for PTSD or MDD, as outlined in the VA/DoD CPGs, in specialty mental health care settings. Providers may be employed in one of three ways: as an active-duty service member (i.e., a uniformed member of the military), as a government civilian employee (i.e., in a General Schedule job), or as a civilian contractor in an MTF (through a contract between the MTF and a private-sector organization).

To understand the characteristics of the PH workforce, we requested data from multiple sources within DoD. The data sources varied depending on whether the provider was an active-duty service member, a civilian, or a DoD contractor. We obtained data on the number and characteristics of active-duty and DoD civilian PH providers from the Defense Manpower Data Center's Health Manpower Personnel Data System (HMPDS). The system does not contain information on contractors, so we requested data on the number and type of contracted PH providers working in MTFs from the Army, Navy, Air Force, and Defense Health Agency (DHA). From each data source, we obtained data for several provider types, including psychiatrists, PNPs, psychologists, social workers, and other master's-level clinicians. In addition to provider type, we obtained information on providers' education level (e.g., master's degree, Ph.D.) and service branch. It should be noted that these data on the PH workforce did not include community providers contracted by the MHS to provide care through the purchased care network. In addition, our data did not include details about the care setting (e.g., inpatient, ambulatory) in which these providers worked. Note that because these data include the entire target population and are not a sample, we did not conduct statistical testing and simply describe the differences observed in these data.

Survey of MTF Psychological Health Providers

This survey was conducted to better understand the capacity of PH providers within MTFs to deliver evidence-based care for PTSD and MDD. Data collected concerned the knowledge, practices, attitudes, and beliefs of PH providers based in MTFs. The survey was administered to a stratified, random sample of PH providers, including psychiatrists (M.D.), PNPs, doctoral-level psychologists, and master's-level clinicians (psychologists or social workers) who had delivered psychiatric treatment (i.e., counseling, psychotherapy, or medication) to adult patients with PTSD or MDD in the past month. The "past month" time frame was selected as an indicator that the provider is currently an active clinician. The sample was limited to behavioral health providers with active-duty or DoD civilian employment status. Civilian contractors were not included because their participation would require Office of Management and Budget (OMB) review and approval under the Paperwork Reduction Act—a regulatory process that can be lengthy. Due to this project's time line, it was not feasible to pursue this approval.

Personnel data from HMPDS provided summary data for targeted PH providers, including license/provider type and service branch. A sample of active-duty and DoD civilian providers (the selection of which is outlined below) was drawn; sampled providers were asked to participate in the study. Of those invited to participate, providers who indicated (through a brief online screening step) that they had treated an adult patient with PTSD or depression in the past month were eligible to complete the full survey.

Sampling Approach

We drew a stratified, random sample of PH providers across MTFs based on provider type, service branch, and employment status. We included four types of providers, including psychiatrists (M.D.), PNPs, doctoral-level psychologists, and master's-level clinicians (psychologists or social workers). We sampled PH providers with active-duty or civilian employee status from Army, Navy,[1] and Air Force. Note that although we stratified our sample on the basis of employment status, we did not take this provider characteristic into account in the analyses presented in this report, as we were not sufficiently powered to detect differences in an additional stratum. Additional details on our sampling approach, including a description of eligible providers in each stratum, are provided in Appendix A.

We designed the sampling approach to allow us to describe the overall population of eligible MTF PH providers, to describe PH providers within each degree type and within each service branch, and to compare providers by degree type and by service branch. To support these analyses, we determined that a final sample of approximately 500 respondents was necessary. We aimed to have a minimum of 50 respondents in each two-dimensional stratum (e.g., Army doctoral-level psychologists), though this objective was constrained somewhat by the breakdown of the provider population across the strata (see Appendix A for details). With

---

[1]   Marine Corps personnel are generally served by PH providers employed by the Navy.

this planned sample, we would be able to detect small to medium effect sizes when comparing provider types and service branches.

To achieve a final survey cohort of 500 respondents, we estimated that we needed to select a sample of approximately 1,500 PH providers. Response rates for provider surveys are typically lower than those for the general population (Kellerman and Herold, 2001). Based on prior research, we assumed that 25 percent of sampled psychiatrists and 45 percent of other providers would respond to the survey. For example, Hawley and colleagues highlighted poor response rates among mental health providers and suggested that typical response rates were between 25 and 40 percent (Hawley, Cook, and Jensen-Doss, 2009).

To be eligible for our survey, a PH provider needed to have seen a patient with PTSD or MDD at an MTF in the previous 30 days. We determined eligibility with a screener item on the survey, as this information was not included in the provider data. We assumed that some sampled providers would not be eligible for the survey. Specifically, we assumed that 50 percent of social workers would not be eligible (based on their response to the screening item regarding providing psychiatric treatment to a patient with PTSD or MDD in the previous month), as many social workers focus on case management and do not provide psychotherapy or medication management. For other provider types, we assumed that all providers would be eligible, as we did not have reliable estimates of the proportion of these providers who solely performed other roles (e.g., administrative duties).

Across the targeted provider types and service branches, there were 3,403 potentially eligible PH providers who had active-duty or government civilian employment status (see Appendix A). We used a stratified, random sampling approach to ensure an adequate number of providers in each provider-type and service stratum based on the assumptions described above.[2] Table 2.1 shows the number of sampled providers in each stratum. We combined psychiatrists and PNPs because there was not an adequate number of PNPs to assess this group on its own and because both of these types of practitioners are often involved in medication management for patients with PTSD or MDD. Further details are provided in Appendix A.

Table 2.1
Sampled Providers, by Provider Type and Service Branch

Provider Type	Total	Army	Navy	Air Force
Total	1,489	657	411	421
Psychiatrists/psychiatric nurse practitioners	536	256	181	99
Psychologists (doctoral level)	349	116	107	126
Master's-level clinicians (master's-level psychologists/ social workers)	604	285	123	196

NOTES: The population includes military and government civilian employee providers who may not be eligible to participate in the survey. The population does not include contractor providers. Eligibility status could be determined only through a survey screener, so the population described in this table includes some ineligible providers.

---

[2] After selecting the initial sample, we determined that 10.4 percent of providers were missing email addresses, required to send survey invitations. We then reselected the sample, limiting eligibility for selection to those providers with email addresses. Final sampling probabilities were adjusted slightly based on the target population with email addresses.

Survey Operations

An experienced survey subcontractor, Davis Research, managed survey administration and data collection. Sampled PH providers were invited to participate via email, followed by mailed invitations to their address of record. Because surveys of health care providers often have low response rates (Kellerman and Herold, 2001; VanGeest, Johnson, and Welch, 2007), we used a mixed-mode strategy to increase the likelihood of higher response rates. Participants had the option to complete the survey online or by telephone. Interviewers contacted nonresponders by telephone and offered to administer the survey via telephone or assist the provider in accessing the survey website. Reminder invitations were sent via regular mail and email.

In total, each potential respondent received up to five email invitations, three hard-copy letters, and 12 telephone calls. Invalid email addresses, telephone numbers, and mailing addresses were removed or updated, when possible, throughout the eight-week survey period, from February to April 2016. Average survey completion time was 19 minutes via web and 45 minutes via phone. Providers who completed the survey during off-duty hours received a $50 gift card. Due to DoD regulations, those who completed the survey during work hours were not eligible to receive an incentive.

Response Rate

Of the 1,489 providers invited to participate, 677 (45.5 percent) accessed the survey and answered the eligibility-screening question. Of these, 22.3 percent (n = 151) were not eligible to complete the survey because they had not provided psychiatric care (i.e., counseling, psychotherapy, or medication management) to an adult patient with PTSD or MDD in the previous 30 days. All of the remaining 526 eligible providers consented to participate. Of 526 providers who completed the survey, 89.2 percent completed the survey via web (n = 469) and 10.8 percent completed the survey via phone (n = 57). The raw response rate was 35.3 percent (526 consented to participate out of 1,489 invited), but this rate does not account for the portion of the sample that we learned was ineligible after selection. Therefore, we computed an adjusted response rate based on published guidelines (American Association for Public Opinion Research, undated, response rate method 2). This rate effectively removed providers eventually deemed ineligible due to either their response on the eligibility-screening item or inaccurate primary contact information (i.e., nonworking email address). This adjusted response rate was 39.3 percent (526 of 1,337). In the process of fielding the survey, we learned that many providers had missing or inaccurate phone numbers. This could be due to the provider leaving the MHS (no longer eligible for the survey), moving to another MTF (still eligible for the survey), or missing data in the sample file. If those in the sample with an inaccurate or unavailable telephone number were removed, the adjusted response rate would be 70.8 percent (526 of 742).

Survey Weighting

Since we did not use simple random sampling (that is, we sampled from some strata with a higher probability than others), and the response rate by provider type was not random (i.e., certain types of providers were more likely to respond than others), we weighted the data to ensure that our analyses represented a relevant population of providers. That is, each provider in our final pool of respondents was assigned a weight calculated as the inverse of the product of that provider's probability of being selected to participate in the study and his or her estimated probability of responding. The design weights were based on service, position title, and military/civilian status, with each respondent assigned one of 30 weights based on these categories, as described earlier. The nonresponse weights were based on a logistic regression model predicting survey response with age, sex, service, an interaction between military/civilian status, and an indicator for a mailing address outside the 50 states. The final weights were the product of the design weight and nonresponse weight. The possibility of trimming the top 1.5 percent of weights was explored but ultimately abandoned due to the very minimal impact on the overall design effect. All analyses incorporated these weights.

Details on our weighting methods are provided in Appendix A. As noted in the appendix, the weighted cohort of respondents is representative of the population of providers eligible for our study. Therefore, when a subgroup of the respondent cohort was analyzed, that subgroup, when weighted using (unmodified) final weights, was representative of the corresponding subgroup of the population of providers. For instance, the weighted set of responding providers that administer psychotherapy was representative of the population of eligible providers that administer psychotherapy.

Final Analytic Sample

Of the 526 responders, six were removed, resulting in a final analytic sample of 520. These providers were removed because their survey responses indicated that they were not an eligible provider type and were sampled in error (registered nurse: n = 3; physiatrist: n = 1) or they did not respond to any items following the eligibility screener (n = 2).

As described earlier, we applied survey weights to enable population estimates. The first two columns in Table 2.2 describe the unweighted final analytic sample. The second two col-

Table 2.2
Final Analytic Sample Compared with the Psychological Health Provider Population

Characteristic	Analytic Sample		Population[b]		Analytic Sample % (weighted)
	N[a]	% (unweighted)	N	%	
Provider type					
Psychiatrist	152	29.2	500	14.7	15.7
Psychiatric nurse practitioner	53	10.2	160	4.7	5.0
Psychologist	139	26.7	1,004	29.5	35.1
Master's-level clinician	176	33.9	1,739	51.1	44.2
Service branch					
Army	203	39.0	2,219	65.2	65.0
Navy	165	31.7	557	16.4	16.3
Air Force	152	29.2	627	18.4	18.7
Military status					
Active duty	317	61.0	1,531	45.0	47.0
Civilian	203	39.0	1,872	55.0	53.1

[a] Total N = 520.

[b] Note that the population includes military and government civilian employee providers who may not be eligible to participate in the study. The population does not include contractor providers. Eligibility status could be determined only through a survey screener, so the population described in this table includes some ineligible providers.

umns describe the population of PH providers from which we drew the sample (see Appendix A for more detail on the full population of providers). The unweighted analytic sample was expected to, and did, differ from the population, because smaller groups (e.g., psychiatrists) were oversampled to ensure adequate power to analyze group differences. The rightmost column describes the final analytic sample after weighting, which largely accounted for differences between the unweighted sample and the population. Note, however, that the population from which we drew the sample includes ineligible providers (since we cannot determine the eligibility status of every provider in this population). Since the analytic sample is weighted to represent the population of only eligible providers, differences between the weighted analytic sample and the population in Table 2.2 are due to the presence of ineligible providers in the population from which we sampled. For example, master's-level clinicians accounted for 44.2 percent of the weighted analytic sample, whereas the population consists of 51.1 percent master's-level clinicians. Likewise, civilians made up 53.1 percent of the weighted sample, but their representation in the population of PH providers is 55 percent. The underrepresentation of master's-level clinicians and civilians in our weighted sample is a consequence of lower eligibility for these providers (i.e., master's-level clinicians and civilian providers were less likely than other provider types to report having treated a patient with MDD or PTSD in the previous 30 days). When reporting all survey results, we present weighted percentages, as the raw numbers are not meaningful.

To account for sampling error, our population-wide estimates had a maximum margin of error of 5.6 percent with survey weights applied. That is, if it is estimated that 50 percent of all providers in our cohort reported engaging in a particular activity, then we can be confident that between 44.4 and 55.6 percent of providers engaged in that activity. Note, too, that the margin of error increases when we calculate values using only certain types of providers, rather than the entire analytic sample. For instance, estimates calculated using only Army providers had a maximum margin of error of 8 percent.

Survey Measures

To select the appropriate measure domains for the survey, we adapted the Consolidated Framework for Implementation Research (Damschroder et al., 2009). Using this model, we considered four domains that could influence the delivery of CPG-recommended care in the MTFs:

1. The **outer setting**, which encompasses the external economic, political, and social influences on an organization (e.g., a specific MTF). For example, federal government budget limitations that can have downstream effects on staffing, provider caseloads, and funding for professional development (e.g., conferences, trainings).
2. The **inner setting**, which includes the structural, political, and social context of an MTF that could govern or influence the use of CPGs. For example,
   a. **Structural characteristics**, such as facility census and provider caseload, which can serve as barriers to CPG adherence, particularly in limited resource settings.
   b. **Implementation climate**, such as the compatibility between the perceived meaning/value of CPGs and the provider's values and needs. This domain also includes peer and leadership support for continued fidelity to evidence-based practice.
   c. **Readiness for implementation** includes leadership engagement, availability of support resources, and ready access to information about CPGs.

3. **Mental health providers**, who are responsible for delivering evidence-based treatment in concordance with CPGs. Characteristics include providers' confidence or self-efficacy in delivering the recommended treatment models and providers' attitudes or beliefs about the appropriateness of the recommended treatment models for their practice and patients.
4. The **implementation processes**, which include communication, training, rules, guidelines, incentives, and disincentives that support or impede delivery of evidence-based, guideline-concordant treatment.

In accordance with the model, we assessed several domains related to the providers, their practice characteristics, and the care they delivered to patients with PTSD and MDD seen in MTFs. Considering that our source of information was a provider survey, within each domain, we included an assessment of those components that are visible to providers and about which they can reliably report. Given this constraint, some components of the Consolidated Framework were not assessed (e.g., federal budget limitations, leadership attitudes). Table 2.3 provides an overview of each domain and the number of items associated with each domain. A more detailed description of the survey domains can be found in Appendix B, and the full survey is available in Appendix C.

Survey Programming

Five screening items were used to appropriately route each provider to survey modules relevant to his or her practice. The first screening item asked whether the respondent had delivered psychiatric treatment (psychotherapy or medication management) to an adult patient with PTSD or MDD in the past 30 days. Only providers who answered "yes" continued with the survey. In other words, all survey results describe a sample of MTF providers active in MDD/PTSD patient care. Providers who worked solely in administrative and/or research roles, and providers who delivered care for other conditions, were not included. The remaining group of active

Table 2.3
Survey Domains and Number of Items

Survey Domain	Topics Assessed in Survey Domain	Domain Question(s) Asked of:	Unweighted Subsample (N)	Number of Items
Eligibility screen: Delivered PTSD/MDD care in past 30 days	Delivery of PTSD and/or MDD care within the past 30 days	All respondents	677	1
Provider attributes				
Provider characteristics	Demographic and professional characteristics	Providers who delivered PTSD or MDD care in the past 30 days	520	6
Theoretical orientation	Primary and secondary theoretical orientation	Providers who delivered PTSD or MDD care in the past 30 days	520	1
Practice attributes				
Practice characteristics	Clinic flow, proportion of patients served with PTSD or MDD	Providers who delivered PTSD or MDD care in the past 30 days	520	8
Measurement-based care	Use of routine, standardized symptom assessments	Providers who delivered PTSD or MDD care in the past 30 days	520	3

Table 2.3—Continued

Survey Domain	Topics Assessed in Survey Domain	Domain Question(s) Asked of:	Unweighted Subsample (N)	Number of Items
Psychotherapy				
Screening items	Whether provider delivered psychotherapy to a PTSD or MDD patient	Providers who delivered PTSD or MDD care in the past 30 days	520	2
Approaches for PTSD	Psychotherapies used to treat PTSD	Providers who delivered PTSD psychotherapy in the past 30 days	404	1
Approaches for MDD	Psychotherapies used to treat MDD	Providers who delivered MDD psychotherapy in the past 30 days	413	1
Techniques for PTSD	Use of guideline-concordant psychotherapy techniques for PTSD	PTSD psychotherapy providers who delivered at least four sessions of psychotherapy to their most recent patient with PTSD	315	19
Techniques for MDD	Use of guideline-concordant psychotherapy techniques for MDD	MDD psychotherapy providers who delivered at least four sessions of psychotherapy to their most recent patient with MDD	310	13
Medication management				
Screening items	Whether provider delivered medication management to a patient with PTSD or MDD	Providers who delivered PTSD or MDD care in the past 30 days	520	2
Medication management for PTSD	Comorbidities and current pharmacological prescriptions for most recent PTSD patient	Providers who delivered PTSD medication management in the past 30 days	186	4
Medication management for MDD	Comorbidities and current pharmacological prescriptions for most recent MDD patient	Providers who delivered MDD medication management in the past 30 days	188	4
Training, supervision, and confidence in guideline-concordant treatments for PTSD and MDD treatment	Hours of training, amount of supervision, and level of confidence for PTSD and MDD treatment	Providers who delivered PTSD or MDD care in the past 30 days	520	27
Barriers to implementing guideline-concordant care	Provider and practice-level barriers to guideline-concordant PTSD and MDD care	Providers who delivered PTSD or MDD care in the past 30 days	520	26
Total Items				118

PTSD/MDD providers answered the modules on provider attributes; practice attributes; training, supervision, and confidence in guideline-concordant treatments; and barriers to implementing guideline-concordant care (Table 2.3).

A series of two screening items assessed whether the respondent had delivered psychological counseling or psychotherapy in the past 30 days to a patient with (1) PTSD or (2) MDD. Only respondents who had delivered psychotherapy to a patient with PTSD in the past 30 days viewed and responded to questions about PTSD psychotherapy approaches and techniques. The program skipped all other providers past these questions. Similarly, only providers who delivered psychotherapy to a patient with MDD in the past 30 days viewed and responded to questions about MDD psychotherapy approaches and techniques. Providers who had delivered psychotherapy to both a PTSD and an MDD patient in the past 30 days received both sections of the questionnaire.

Finally, two screening items assessed whether the respondent had prescribed a medication or delivered a medication management visit in the past 30 days to a patient with (1) PTSD or (2) MDD. Similar to the logic above, only providers who actively provided medication management services viewed and responded to questions about medication management. The survey was programmed to skip all other providers past these questions. Providers who had delivered medication management to both a PTSD and an MDD patient in the past 30 days received both sections of the questionnaire.

Data Analyses

We conducted descriptive analyses to examine survey-weighted means, frequencies, and conditional crosstabs. We evaluated subgroup differences by provider type and service branch in means, proportions, and frequencies for continuous and binary outcomes using Wald tests of coefficients from survey-weighted generalized linear models. We assessed subgroup differences in categorical outcomes using F-statistics from survey-weighted contingency tables. All reported p-values were adjusted for multiple comparisons within each survey domain using the false discovery rate method (Benjamini and Hochberg, 1995). Although an analysis of service branch by provider type would have provided useful information, the cell sizes were such that we lacked the power to pursue tests of the interaction between service branch and provider type. Therefore, all analyses that follow describe main effects of provider type and service branch separately.

Key Informant Discussions

To understand the context within the MHS with respect to promoting and monitoring the quality of PH care, we conducted semi-structured discussions with individuals knowledgeable about PH care delivery within the MHS. Key informant interviews were completed during the same time frame as the fielding of the survey of MTF providers.

Selection of Key Informants

We selected key informants according to their position and responsibilities within the MHS. All participants had duties related to the oversight, structure, and delivery of PH care. To ensure diverse representation of personnel across the MHS, we invited a total of 12 stakeholders from DHA, DCoE, the Office of the Assistant Secretary of Defense for Health Affairs (OASD/HA), and each of the four service branches (Army, Navy, Air Force, and Marine Corps) to participate. Invitations were sent by email. Of those originally invited, two declined to participate and one did not respond despite several follow-up emails. For one of the discussions, a key informant invited additional colleagues to participate. All told, a total of 11 individuals participated in nine discussion sessions. Therefore, the breakdown of stakeholders participation by organization was as follows: DCoE (1); DHA (4); Army (2); Navy (2); Air Force (1); Marine Corps (1).

Discussion Domains

Key informants provided insights about PH care within the MHS as it related to their official roles and responsibilities. Discussions focused on three major areas: (1) organization of the PH workforce, (2) utilization management and performance measurement, and (3) quality-improvement efforts for PH care. The discussion guide is included in Appendix D. Discussions were conducted via telephone, and each discussion lasted between 45 and 60 minutes. A RAND researcher led the discussions, and a second member of the RAND research team took notes.

Analyses

We reviewed discussion notes to identify and group responses by themes relevant to our study aims. In addition to organizing the information by theme, we noted differences in PH organization across military branches and highlighted the unique challenges each branch faced in ensuring high-quality PH care for service members. Furthermore, we noted the various mechanisms for performance monitoring and quality improvement that had been implemented across different military settings. Findings and insights from these discussions are woven into our presentation of findings in the chapters that follow.

CHAPTER THREE

Characteristics of the Psychological Health Workforce Across the MHS

The MHS provides health care services to active-duty and retired military personnel and their dependents. It is a complex organization, with care provided directly in MTFs by the service branches (Air Force, Army, and Navy, which provides Marine Corps care) and purchased in the community through TRICARE, DoD's health benefits program. OASD/HA issues guidance and regulations related to health care policy and oversees the management of DoD medical programs, though the service branches develop and issue service-specific health care policies as well. DHA was established in 2013 to improve integration, standardization, and quality of care across the MHS. It is responsible for managing the implementation of OASD/HA-issued policies across the service branches, monitoring outcomes and quality of care, and increasing the use of evidence-based health care practices across the MHS.

Although OASD/HA and DHA guide MHS policy direction and implementation, the responsibility to recruit, organize, train, and fund medical personnel belongs to the three service branches. Additionally, the majority of the MTFs and clinics that deliver health care services fall under the medical command structures of the individual branches (U.S. Government Accountability Office, 2015). As such, the organization and delivery of health care—and particularly PH care—varies widely by service branch. In the next section, we describe the PH workforce across MTFs, noting differences by service branch and provider type. We also provide an overview of how psychological care services are configured within the service branches. We do not describe the organization of PH care across the MHS in detail; this was not the focus of our project and has been addressed elsewhere (Department of Defense, 2014; Hoge et al., 2015; Quaadgras, Glasmeier, and Kaplan, 2016).

In this report, we focus on a subset of all PH provider types—namely, psychiatrists, PNPs, doctoral-level psychologists, and master's-level clinicians (psychologists and social workers). Although MTFs are staffed with substance abuse counselors, mental health nurses, and other providers involved in care for PTSD or MDD, we focused on those specialty PH provider types most likely to be responsible for delivering formal, guideline-recommended treatments (i.e., psychopharmacologic medication, psychotherapy) for these conditions. In addition, while we acknowledge the important role of primary care providers in treating PTSD and MDD (particularly in delivering medication treatment), we did not include these providers, as the focus of our research was on specialty PH providers. We did include specialty PH providers who work in primary care, however, and we describe how PH care is delivered in both primary and specialty care settings.

Service Branch Differences in the Size and Composition of the Psychological Health Workforce

The MHS employs almost 4,000 psychiatrists, PNPs, psychologists, and social workers at MTFs. Table 3.1 shows the number of PH providers by provider type and service branch.

The Army PH workforce is almost three times larger than that of the Air Force or Navy, reflecting the size of the Army relative to the other services. In 2016, the total number of active-duty Army personnel was 474,000, while the Navy had 330,000, the Marine Corps had 184,000, and the Air Force had 314,000 (Defense Manpower Data Center, 2016). At the population level, the Army has a ratio of PH providers to active-duty personnel more than twice as high as the other services, with 4.7 PH providers per 1,000 active-duty soldiers, compared with 1.7 PH providers per 1,000 active-duty sailors and Marines for the Navy and 2.6 PH providers per 1,000 active-duty airmen for the Air Force. The relative size of the Army PH workforce appears to reflect the higher proportions of soldiers receiving PH treatment compared with airmen, Marines, and sailors. In a recent study on the quality of PH care in the MHS (Hepner et al., 2017), Army personnel represented nearly 70 percent of an identified cohort of service members who received a diagnosis of PTSD in 2013, while Navy, Marine Corps, and Air Force personnel each accounted for approximately 10 percent.

Overall, master's-level clinicians made up almost half (48 percent) of the PH provider workforce; most of them are social workers (94 percent), with a small number of civilian master's-level psychologists also employed (6 percent). A third of the overall PH workforce is doctoral-level psychologists, though this proportion is greater in the Air Force (42 percent) and Navy (40 percent) than in the Army (27 percent). Psychiatrists make up a greater proportion of the Navy's PH workforce (22 percent) than in the Air Force (12 percent) or Army (14 percent).

The military departments have a number of mechanisms for employing PH providers. Some PH providers are active-duty military, some are civilian government employees, and some are contractors; the proportion of each differs by service (Table 3.2). Contractors make up more than a third of the Navy's PH workforce but less than 10 percent of the Army's. Two-thirds of the Air Force PH workforce is uniformed personnel, compared with 27 percent in the Army workforce and 37 percent in the Navy. The majority (67 percent) of Army mental health providers are civilian employees.

Table 3.1
Composition of Military Treatment Facility Psychological Health Provider Workforce, by Provider Type and Service Branch

Service Branch	Total Providers	Psychiatrists		PNPs		Doctoral-Level Psychologists		Master's-Level Clinicians	
		N	%	N	%	N	%	N	%
Army	2,365	320	14	89	4	638	27	1,318	56
Navy	892	193	22	67	8	354	40	278	31
Air Force	830	96	12	31	4	350	42	353	43
DoD total	4,131	612	15	189	5	1,358	33	1,972	48

NOTES: Total DoD numbers include 44 PH providers employed by the DHA National Capital Region Medical Directorate. Master's-level clinicians include both master's-level psychologists and social workers.

Table 3.2
Composition of the Psychological Health Provider Workforce, by Employment Type and Service Branch

Service Branch	Total Providers	Active-Duty Military (%)	Civilian (%)	Contractor (%)
Army	2,365	27	67	6
Navy	892	37	25	38
Air Force	830	67	8	24
DoD total	4,131	37	45	18

NOTES: The DHA National Capital Region Medical Directorate (including Walter Reed National Military Medical Center and other joint service medical installations) employs an additional 44 PH providers as contractors, who are not reflected in the table. The Army contractor data we received collapsed master's- and doctoral-level psychologists (n = 48); based on patterns in the data for other services, we categorized all these providers as doctoral-level psychologists.

Although these data provide important insights about the size and nature of the PH workforce at MTFs, it is worth noting that some providers may not treat patients. Some of these providers may predominantly or solely perform administrative duties. We were unable to assess current practice locations with the available data.

Organization of MTF PH Provider Workforce
Although each service branch develops its own processes and policies for recruiting, hiring, and staffing its PH workforce, DoD provides guidance and tools for doing so. One example is the Psychological Health Risk Adjustment Model for Staffing, a clinic-level model for determining the optimal staff mix across provider types, given the prevalence of PH conditions in the local population and other population characteristics (U.S. Government Accountability Office, 2015). Each MTF typically has a mix of psychiatrists, PNPs, doctoral- and master's-level psychologists, and clinical social workers based in specialty mental health care clinics, though key differences by service branch are described by our key informant discussions.

The Army has taken an innovative approach to PH provider staffing. Historically, the PH provider workforce was divided by discipline into departments (e.g., psychology, social work). However, in 2010, the Army reorganized its staffing structure to deliver what it perceived to be more sustainable, cost-effective, standardized care to soldiers and their dependents. Army PH care is now provided through 12 structured programs with an integrated mix of PH personnel from diverse disciplinary backgrounds, including psychology, psychiatry, psychiatric nursing, and social work (Hoge et al., 2015).[1] At the installation level, each integrated PH department is supervised by a clinical chief.

Navy MTFs are staffed according to population needs; the Navy's Bureau of Medicine works with subject-matter experts from each provider discipline to determine the PH staffing mix at each MTF. Each Navy MTF is staffed with at least one psychiatrist and one doctoral-

---

[1]   The 12 programs are Behavioral Health in Patient Centered Medical Homes, Child and Family Behavioral Health System, Family Advocacy Program, Behavioral Health in Soldier Centered Medical Homes, Embedded Behavioral Health, Multidisciplinary Behavioral Health Services, Intensive Outpatient Programs, Inpatient Behavioral Health Services, Residential Treatment Facilities, Connect Care, Tele-Behavioral Health, and the Behavioral Health Data Portal (BHDP). In the Army, Patient Centered Medical Homes deliver care for families of active-duty soldiers, while Soldier Centered Medical Homes are specifically for soldiers.

level psychologist. The Navy and the Marine Corps work collaboratively to deliver PH care to Marine Corps personnel. In most cases, Navy providers are stationed at Marine Corps bases but work in Navy-operated MTFs; these providers report to Navy leadership at these MTFs, as well as to the Navy Surgeon General. Some Navy providers are attached to Marine Corps operational units and are under the command and credentialing authority of the Marine Corps.

In the Air Force, all MTFs are staffed with a psychologist and a social worker, but only large and medium MTFs have a psychiatrist; for smaller MTFs, treatment from a psychiatrist is available via telehealth. In some cases, psychiatric care is delivered through the purchased care network; the network is viewed as an extension of Air Force psychological health care capacity.

Across the MHS, there have been multiple efforts to integrate PH providers into primary care settings. The Army has undertaken the most extensive of these efforts. In Army primary care clinics, licensed PH providers provide support through expert consultations, clinical assessments, triage, and brief cognitive behavioral interventions (Hoge et al., 2015). Integrating PH in this way has improved access and continuity of care, as well as enhanced communication among primary care providers, PH providers, and unit leaders (Hoge et al., 2015). Navy Medicine has also integrated PH providers into the primary care setting and into line units. Integrated Navy PH consultants are housed in primary care settings to provide consultation and deliver short-term care to patients. Similarly, the Air Force has implemented a program to embed behavioral health providers into primary care delivery. These providers deliver short-term care focused on education, skill building, self-management, and home-based strategies (Air Force Medical Service, 2013).

Individual and Practice Characteristics of Surveyed MTF PH Providers

As described in Chapter Two, we surveyed a representative sample of uniformed and civilian PH providers across MTFs, which allowed us to describe additional characteristics of the MTF PH provider workforce not included in existing data. While survey respondents were weighted to reflect the overall population of providers (psychiatrists, PNPs, psychologists, and master's-level clinicians), service branches (Air Force, Army, and Navy), and military status (active-duty or DoD civilian) within MTFs (see Table 2.2), the survey sample was different from the overall population of PH providers in that it did not include contracted providers, who constitute 18 percent of the overall PH workforce (and 38 percent of the Navy PH workforce).

After applying the survey weights, master's-level clinicians (44 percent) made up the largest proportion of providers who completed the survey, followed by psychologists (35 percent). Army providers represented nearly two-thirds of respondents, and respondents were approximately evenly split between active-component and DoD civilian providers.[2]

Individual PH Provider Characteristics

On average, surveyed PH providers had been practicing for 13.8 years (standard error [SE] = 0.55). The majority of providers were white (70.5 percent), while 7.5 percent were Hispanic, 5.8 percent were black or African American, 5.3 percent were Asian, 1.6 percent were Ameri-

---

[2]   Only active-duty and civilian government employee PH providers were invited to complete the survey due to regulatory requirements. As described earlier, contracted providers make up 18 percent of the overall PH workforce.

can Indian or Alaska Native, 4.2 percent were multiple races, and 5.2 percent identified with a different category (i.e., Native Hawaiian or other Pacific Islander, other, and unknown).

Theoretical Orientation

Theoretical orientation is an overall framework to guide how a provider approaches conceptualizing and treating patients (Poznanski and McLennan, 1995; Ogunfowora and Drapeau, 2008). Theoretical orientation is typically directly related to type of treatments that the provider delivers (e.g., providers with a cognitive therapeutic orientation typically deliver cognitive behavioral therapy), but they are separate concepts. When asked to endorse a primary theoretical orientation, nearly half of providers selected cognitive (48.5 percent), followed by behavioral (10.2 percent), as shown in Figure 3.1.

Theoretical orientations varied across provider types (Table 3.3). The majority of master's-level clinicians and doctoral-level psychologists indicated that their primary theoretical orientation was cognitive. Both groups were significantly more likely to endorse a cognitive orientation than were psychiatrists/PNPs ($ps < 0.001$). Consistent with their role as prescribers, psychiatrists/PNPs were most likely to select biological as their primary theoretical orientation and were significantly more likely to do so than were behavioral providers ($ps < 0.001$). Endorsement of a biological theoretical orientation was the only orientation item that differed across service branches ($p < 0.01$). Navy providers (16.5 percent) were more likely than both Army (6.5 percent, $p < 0.001$) and Air Force providers (6.2 percent, $p < 0.05$) to select biological as their primary theoretical orientation. Given that psychiatrists made up a greater proportion of the PH workforce in the Navy than in the Army and Air Force, a greater endorsement of a biological orientation in the Navy is unsurprising.

Figure 3.1
Endorsed Primary Theoretical Orientation Among Providers Who Delivered PTSD or MDD Services in the Past 30 Days

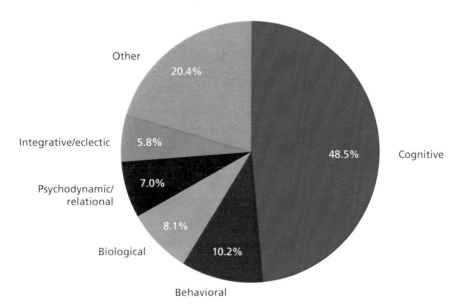

NOTES: n = 517. "Other" includes Rogerian/person-centered, humanistic, existential, interpersonal, psychoanalytic, experiential/gestalt, acceptance/third wave, and systems/family systems.
RAND RR1692-3.1

Table 3.3
Percentage Who Endorsed Each Primary Theoretical Orientation, Among Providers Who Delivered PTSD or MDD Services in the Past 30 Days, by Provider Type

Orientation	Master's-Level Clinicians	Doctoral-Level Psychologists	Psychiatrists/ PNPs	American Psychological Association Psychotherapy Division (2012)
Cognitive***	58.6[a]	53.1[a]	18.9[b]	17
Behavioral	11.8	7.9	10.9	3
Biological***	0.4[a]	0.3[a]	37.9[b]	—
Psychodynamic/relational	5.1	5.3	14.1	27
Integrative/eclectic*	2.1[a]	10.6[b]	5.5[a,b]	25
Acceptance/third wave***	0.3[a]	12.5[b]	1.7[a]	—
Systems/family systems	5.8	1.0	1.0	2
Other	22.0	22.8	12.7	26

SOURCE: American Psychological Association data from a 2012 survey of psychotherapy providers reported in Norcross and Rogan, 2013.
NOTES: n = 513. Values with differing superscripts within rows are significantly different at the $p < 0.05$ level based on post hoc paired comparisons using Wald tests for binary and continuous variables and F statistics for categorical outcomes.
* $p < 0.05$, ** $p < 0.01$, *** $p < 0.001$ for omnibus tests.

The theoretical orientation item was modified from a survey that the Psychotherapy Division of the American Psychological Association used to assess its members, overwhelmingly doctoral-level psychologists (Norcross and Rogan, 2013). The last column in Table 3.3 provides useful data against which to compare military psychologists. Military psychologists appeared to endorse a cognitive orientation (53 percent) at a higher rate than the civilian psychologists who were members of the American Psychological Association's psychotherapy division (17 percent; Norcross and Rogan, 2013). They also appear to be less likely to endorse a psychodynamic or integrative/eclectic orientation. Given a theoretical alignment between a cognitive orientation and evidence-based treatments, such as cognitive behavioral therapy and cognitive processing therapy, this may indicate that military psychologists are more aligned with and likely to provide evidence-based care relative to their civilian counterparts.

In Table 3.3 and others in the report, superscripts are used to indicate significant group differences within table rows. For example, the first row of Table 3.3 shows group differences in the percentage of providers who indicated that their primary theoretical orientation was cognitive. Master's-level clinicians and doctoral-level psychologists have the same superscript (a), which signifies that these groups were not significantly different from one another. However, psychiatrists/PNPs have a different superscript, (b), which signifies that the percentage of psychiatrists/PNPs who endorsed the item was significantly different from the other two groups. The American Psychological Association Psychotherapy Division results were published in aggregate, and therefore, we are unable to compute the pairwise comparisons for this group.

Practice Characteristics

Recall that all eligible respondents indicated that they had provided clinical services to at least one adult patient with PTSD or MDD in the past 30 days. That is, all respondents in the sample are active clinicians. Providers reported having an average of 23 patient visits (adults and children) per week at an MTF. Master's-level clinicians and psychologists reported significantly fewer visits per week (21) than psychiatrists/PNPs (29 visits/week; Table 3.4). Given that psychotherapy sessions are typically scheduled for 45 to 60 minutes and medication management visits are 15 to 30 minutes, this difference in the number of weekly sessions across provider types should be expected. In addition, these average weekly caseloads are comparable to those reported by civilian psychiatrists (33.2 visits/week) and civilian psychologists (21.7 visits/week) (Pingitore et al., 2002).

Providers reported that approximately one-quarter of visits occurred in a primary care setting, though this differed by provider type (Table 3.4). Specifically, master's-level clinicians reported having significantly more patient visits in a primary care setting than did psychologists and psychiatrists/PNPs ($ps < 0.05$).

On their own, patients with PTSD or MDD did not represent the majority of providers' current caseloads. Across all providers, most indicated that less than a quarter of their current patients had PTSD. Similarly, most providers reported that less than a quarter of their current patients had MDD. There were no provider-type differences in the percentage of patients with either of these conditions.

Table 3.4
Practice Characteristics Among Providers Who Delivered PTSD or MDD Services in the Past 30 Days, by Provider Type

Characteristic	All Providers	Master's-Level Clinicians	Doctoral-Level Psychologists	Psychiatrists/ PNPs
Average number of patient visits per week (SE)***	22.6 (0.6)	21.0 (1.0)[a]	20.8 (0.9)[a]	28.9 (1.1)[b]
Percentage of visits in primary care setting (SE)***	24.0 (0.3)	35.0 (0.5)[a]	18.9 (0.4)[b]	9.9 (0.2)[b]
Current patients with PTSD (%)				
None	1.8	2.0	2.3	0.7
1–25	59.0	60.8	57.0	58.5
26–50	28.8	25.2	32.3	30.6
> 50	10.4	12.0	8.5	10.2
Current patients with MDD (%)				
None	1.8	1.7	2.8	0.3
1–25	61.8	66.5	64.5	47.2
26–50	27.3	25.8	22.6	38.6
> 50	9.1	6.0	10.2	13.9

NOTES: N = 520. Values with differing superscripts within rows are significantly different at the $p < 0.05$ level based on post hoc paired comparisons using Wald tests for binary and continuous variables and F statistics for categorical outcomes.

***Omnibus test $p < 0.001$.

Table 3.5
Practice Characteristics by Service Branch, Among Providers Who Delivered PTSD or MDD Services in the Past 30 Days

Characteristic	Army	Navy	Air Force
Average number of patient visits per week (SE)***	22.8 (0.85)[a]	27.0 (1.03)[b]	18.2 (0.72)[c]
Percentage of visits in primary care setting (SE)**	29.1 (3.86)[a]	17.0 (2.94)[b]	12.2 (2.63)[b]
Current patients with PTSD (%)***	[a]	[b]	[b]
None	55.4	62.7	68.4
1–25	31.2	26.9	22.1
26–50	13.2	7.5	3.2
> 50	0.2	3.0	6.4
Current patients with MDD (%)			
None	64.4	53.8	59.7
1–25	25.4	32.8	29.2
26–50	8.8	13.0	6.8
> 50	1.4	0.4	4.3

NOTES: N = 520. Values with differing superscripts within rows are significantly different at the $p < 0.05$ level based on post hoc paired comparisons using Wald tests for binary and continuous variables and F statistics for categorical outcomes.
**$p < 0.01$, ***$p < 0.001$ for omnibus tests.

There were also significant differences in practice characteristics across service branches (Table 3.5). Navy providers saw significantly more patients each week than Army providers who, in turn, saw more patients than Air Force providers. The Navy's provider mix includes a higher proportion of psychiatrists (see Table 3.1), so the shorter visit times and higher caseloads among psychiatrists likely explain the Navy differences, but it is unclear why Army providers have more patient visits per week than Air Force providers.

There were also differences with respect to setting. Army providers saw a greater proportion of their patients in primary care settings than did Air Force and Navy providers. This finding may be attributable to extensive Army efforts to increase integration of PH and primary care (Hoge et al., 2015). Army providers' caseloads had more patients with PTSD, consistent with research showing that members of the Army are more likely than members of the Air Force and Navy to develop PTSD (Schell and Marshall, 2008). The percentage of providers' caseloads made up of patients with MDD was not significantly different by service branch.

Summary

The MTF PH workforce is composed of multiple provider types (Table 3.1). Master's-level clinicians, including master's-level psychologists (3 percent) and social workers (45 percent), make up the largest sector of the workforce (48 percent). While doctoral-level psychologists make up one-third of the workforce, psychiatrists and PNPs represent a smaller portion

(20 percent). There are differences in workforce composition by service; the Air Force, for example, has a higher proportion of doctoral-level psychologists (42 percent) than the Army (27 percent). Most MTF PH providers are active-duty service members (37 percent) or civilian government employees (45 percent). While contractors constitute a relatively small portion of the overall MTF PH workforce (18 percent), this also varies by service. For instance, contractors make up 38 percent of the PH workforce in the Navy but only 6 percent in the Army.

On average, surveyed PH providers had been practicing for 14 years. When compared with civilian psychologists, a larger proportion of surveyed MTF doctoral-level psychologists endorsed theoretical orientations associated with evidence-based psychotherapies (i.e., cognitive and behavioral orientations (Table 3.3). This comparison provides preliminary, but promising, evidence that military psychologists may be more aligned with evidence-based care relative to their civilian counterparts.

Overall, surveyed PH providers reported seeing approximately 23 patients per week (Table 3.4). While psychologists averaged 21 patients per week, psychiatrists/PNPs reported an average of 29 patients per week. These caseloads are comparable to those of civilian psychologists and psychiatrists (21.7 and 33.2 visits per week, respectively). One-fourth of surveyed PH providers reported treating patients in a primary care setting. The majority of providers reported that patients with PTSD or MDD each made up less than 25 percent of their caseload.

CHAPTER FOUR

Delivery of Guideline-Concordant Care for PTSD and MDD

In this chapter, we begin by summarizing findings from our key informant discussions, which provided an overview of how the MHS and the individual services monitor the use of guideline-concordant care. This provides important backdrop for understanding how, at a system level, individual provider performance contributes to the overall quality of PH care delivered at MTFs. Following this overview, we use survey data to describe provider self-reported use of guideline-concordant psychotherapy and medication management for PTSD and MDD, as well as the extent to which providers reported using standardized instruments to measure patient outcomes and adjust treatment plans (measurement-based care).

Approaches to Monitoring Provider Performance and Use of Guideline-Concordant Care

Because the service branches are responsible for their own PH workforces, they are largely responsible for assessing and monitoring the performance of their PH providers and the extent to which providers use CPG-recommended treatments. The service branches run their health care delivery systems largely independently, so these mechanisms can differ widely across branches. In an effort to standardize the assessment of PH care delivery across MTFs, in 2013, the Assistant Secretary of Defense for Health Affairs released a memorandum ordering the service branches to implement the BHDP. BHDP is an Army-originated web-based tool that uses validated instruments to capture clinical mental health outcomes (Woodson, 2013).

Army

In 2012, Army developed BHDP to monitor quality of care and assess provider performance. It is an easy-to-use, secure, web-based system for collecting behavioral health symptom data directly from patients seen in MTFs and has been in operation in Army behavioral health clinics since September 2013 (Hoge et al., 2015). The system is separate from patients' electronic health records. Symptom questionnaires (e.g., the nine-item Patient Health Questionnaire, PTSD Checklist) are collected at treatment initiation and then at follow-up visits. Patients are prompted to complete the questionnaire after the provider manually enters the patient's information and selects the appropriate diagnosis. BHDP data can be used to assess quality of care at the patient-provider level and on a population health scale. Individual providers can use the data to provide patient feedback and adjust treatment based on clinical progress. Patient-level data can be aggregated at the MTF, regional, and Army Health System levels to provide a population perspective on PH outcomes. Furthermore, these aggregate data can provide a nuanced understanding of variations in clinical outcomes by multiple variables, including MTF, race, gender, and baseline symptom assessment score.

The Army also uses BHDP data for quality assessment by measuring specific processes of care. Army leadership emphasizes that patients with PTSD or MDD should receive a minimally adequate number of visits within a specified amount of time (e.g., four sessions within 90 days of diagnosis) and monitors whether MTFs are meeting this goal. The Army also uses BHDP data as part of a value-based incentive system, which incentivizes high performance at the MTF level. Under this system, MTFs are rewarded for both productivity and outcomes. For example, MTFs can receive up to $500 for each soldier who achieves clinical response or remission.

Assessment data are communicated to providers and other stakeholders in multiple ways. First, BHDP data are available to Army leadership across provider types. Information on clinical outcome performance rates is reported by MTFs internally and can be further aggregated at the regional or Army Health System level. Feedback about provider productivity is delivered through the Capacity Assessment and Reporting Tool, which details the monthly performance of every Army provider (by name) and is available for every provider to view. The Army believes this fosters transparency, as well as healthy competition among providers. The Army also communicates performance assessment findings to DoD through its participation in the Mental Health Strategic Work Group, which works to streamline PH care across the services.

Navy and Marine Corps

Prior to the mandate for BHDP implementation, the Navy assessed the quality of its PH care via Psychological Health Pathways, a program that aimed to improve the quality and coordination of PH care through standardized processes for clinical patient assessment, data management, and reporting (Naval Center for Combat and Operational Stress Control, undated-b). However, like the other services, the Navy is now implementing BHDP across all of its MTFs (Naval Center for Combat and Operational Stress Control, undated-a). The Navy began BHDP implementation after the release of a memorandum from then–Assistant Secretary of Defense Jonathan Woodson that mandated implementation across all service branches (Woodson, 2013).

The Navy Psychological Health Advisory Board conducts quality assessment checks by examining compliance with CPGs for specific disorders. To assess compliance rates at MTFs, the group reviews patient charts for particular processes, such as offers of evidence-based psychotherapy, suicide assessment, and appropriate medication use. It also tracks avoidance of contraindicated medications, as well as prescriptions for appropriate medications for PTSD. Findings are communicated to MTFs with high compliance rates to identify best practices and to MTFs with lower compliance rates to better understand reasons for poor performance.

The Marine Corps is in the process of executing plans to measure care through a number of top-down and bottom-up strategies. For example, the Marine Corps Psychological Health Advisory Council, a newly created top-down mechanism, will oversee integral aspects of PH care in the Marine Corps. Its strategic plan involves six lines of effort:

1. integration at the installation and unit levels
2. creation of doctrine, training, and other structural pieces to organize Navy PH providers under Marine Corps command
3. increased focus on suicide

4. increased focus on metrics and performance measures
5. the development and implementation of a PH research agenda
6. increased focus on Marine Corps reservist health.

Bottom-up strategies to be implemented include the creation of goals and metrics for use in the field and the collection of best practices from Marine Expeditionary Forces.

Air Force

In the Air Force, provider performance is most often assessed through peer review. This is a required process for all providers, irrespective of rank. Approximately 10 percent of a provider's records are reviewed, and those with fewer patients often have a higher proportion of their caseload reviewed. Reviewers use templates to ensure that particular clinical processes are covered and that a given diagnosis matches information in the chart notes. Providers receive feedback on their performance via written communication or in-person meetings. This feedback serves as a type of supervision and consultation service, and it is designed to ensure that appropriate care is delivered. High-interest cases, in which patients have numerous risk factors, such as documented suicide risk or visits to multiple types of mental health centers (e.g., substance abuse and family advocacy clinics), are very closely monitored. The Air Force is also implementing BHDP across its MTFs. In November 2015, the Secretary of the Air Force released instructions on BHDP use for clinical outcome tracking and communicating mental health information during patient transfer or termination (U.S. Department of the Air Force, 2015). At the time of this writing, the Air Force had not yet fully implemented BHDP and was not using the data to monitor/assess process of care outcomes.

BHDP Implementation

While several key informants understood that BHDP would be a means of improving the quality of PH care MHS-wide, Navy and Air Force informants noted several implementation challenges that impeded this progress. One participant cited the logistical and technical challenges associated with physical implementation of the platform at every MTF across the country, given the variation across clinics nationwide and the necessary change in business operations. Others discussed the multiple costs associated with the change, including time and technology costs. They added that many clinics would have to be restructured to accommodate the platform. Cultural resistance was also noted as a challenge: Obtaining buy-in from the services, providers, and patients to use BHDP in the most effective way would require a political shift and a willingness to change. Additionally, key informants noted a lack of guidance on *how* BHDP implementation should occur, stating that this increased the difficulty of adopting the platform. Despite these challenges, the implementation of BHDP across MTFs is expected to centralize and increase the visibility of efforts to monitor quality of care and outcomes. At the time of this writing, DHA was working with the service branches to feed BHDP data into the Health Services Data Warehouse, a central repository of clinical and health care delivery data that is used for quality monitoring and reporting, clinical decision support, health care planning, surveillance, research, and other purposes.

Now that we have outlined the general approaches to assessing and monitoring the quality of PH care across the MHS, we turn to the results from our survey that provide detail on the extent to which providers at MTFs deliver guideline-concordant care. These results are organized by the type of clinical approach: delivery of psychotherapy, medication management, and use of measurement-based care.

Delivery of Guideline-Concordant Psychotherapy

Psychotherapy Approaches for PTSD

Our provider survey included a comprehensive list of 30 psychotherapy approaches that could be used with a PTSD patient (see Appendix C, item PTSD1 for the complete list). Embedded in the list were the four psychotherapies that the VA/DoD CPG for posttraumatic stress explicitly identifies as grade-A psychotherapies for PTSD (i.e., cognitive processing therapy, prolonged exposure, eye movement desensitization and reprocessing, and stress inoculation training). Cognitive behavioral therapy that is not "trauma-focused" is identified in the CPG as "less effective." Although the survey's list of psychotherapies included cognitive behavioral therapy, we did not include trauma-focused cognitive behavioral therapy as a treatment option. Finally, the list included additional psychotherapies not identified as "effective treatments" in the VA/DoD CPG. Survey respondents indicated psychotherapies that they have ever used to treat a patient with PTSD and were then asked to select their "primary mode of therapy" for treating PTSD.[1] This section of the survey was limited to respondents who had provided psychotherapy to at least one patient with PTSD in the previous 30 days. Of the total 520 respondents, 404 (77.7 percent) indicated that they had done so.

Across all psychotherapy providers, the most frequently endorsed primary psychotherapy approach was cognitive processing therapy, followed by cognitive behavioral therapy and prolonged exposure (Figure 4.1). We created a composite of the percentage of providers who selected *any* of the VA/DoD CPG-endorsed, grade-A PTSD psychotherapies as their primary psychotherapy approach (i.e., cognitive processing therapy, prolonged exposure, eye movement desensitization and reprocessing, or stress inoculation training) and found that more than half of providers (59.1 percent) selected at least one of these psychotherapies. We excluded cognitive behavioral therapy from this combination because we could not be certain whether it was trauma-focused, as recommended by the VA/DoD CPG.[2] This number would increase to 78.8 percent if we assumed that providers deliver only *trauma-focused* cognitive behavioral therapy as their primary approach for patients with PTSD.

This composite variable for providers who selected any CPG-endorsed psychotherapy for PTSD as their primary approach differed significantly across provider types ($p < 0.001$). Psychologists (77.7 percent) were more likely than master's-level clinicians (55.7 percent, $p < 0.01$), who were more likely than psychiatrists/PNPs (21.3 percent, $p < 0.001$) to select a VA/ DoD CPG-identified effective treatment for PTSD as their primary psychotherapy approach for patients with PTSD. Among psychiatrists and PNPs who delivered psychotherapy, one-fifth relied on guideline-concordant, grade-A psychotherapies for patients with PTSD. That said, a substantial number (16.6 percent) endorsed "supportive counseling" as their primary mode

---

[1] Providers could select any treatment as their "primary mode" or indicate that they had "ever used" each treatment. They were not required to indicate that they had received training or supervision in these psychotherapies to select them.

[2] The rate at which master's-level clinicians, doctoral-level psychologists, and psychiatrists selected cognitive behavioral therapy as their primary therapy did not differ significantly from one another.

Figure 4.1
Primary Psychotherapy Approach for PTSD Among Providers Who Delivered Psychotherapy for PTSD in the Past 30 Days

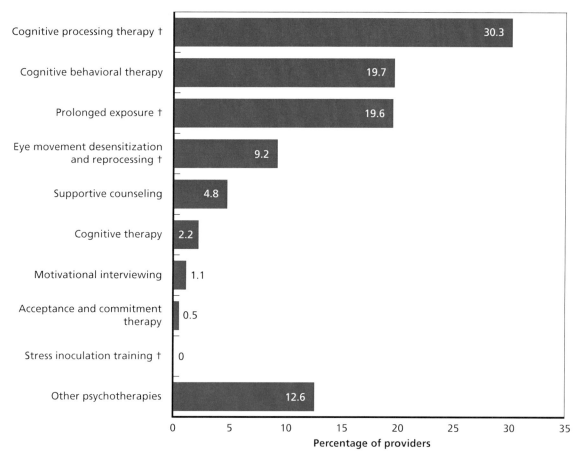

Percentage of providers

NOTES: n = 404. † = Psychotherapies identified as recommended treatments for PTSD in the VA/DoD CPG for that condition. The category "Other psychotherapies" includes dialectical behavioral therapy, integrative/eclectic, behavioral therapy/behavioral activation, psychoanalysis, reality therapy, seeking safety, interpersonal therapy, time limited psychodynamic therapy, Rogerian or other client-centered approach, existential therapy, traditional psychodynamic therapy, hypnosis, and problem solving therapy.
RAND RR1692-4.1

for PTSD, suggesting that they may have reported on therapy provided as an adjunct to medication management (rather than a stand-alone psychotherapy). If we were to assume that all supportive counseling selected by psychiatrists/PNPs was an appropriate adjunct to medication management, then the rate of guideline-concordant psychotherapy would rise among psychiatrists/PNPs from 21.3 percent to 37.9 percent. Unfortunately, we are unable to determine this based on the survey responses. Aside from these composite differences, the primary psychotherapy modes used to treat PTSD also varied across provider types (Table 4.1).

There were significant differences across service branches related to the specific primary psychotherapy approach delivered to patients with PTSD (Table 4.2). There was also a service branch difference in the composite variable assessing the percentage of providers who selected *any* of the VA/DoD grade-A psychotherapies for PTSD as their primary approach ($p < 0.001$). PH providers in the Air Force (79.6 percent) were significantly more likely than providers in the Army (54.7 percent, $p < 0.001$) and Navy (54.1 percent, $p < 0.001$) to select a primary

Table 4.1
Primary Psychotherapy Approach for PTSD Among Providers Who Delivered Psychotherapy for PTSD in the Past 30 Days, by Provider Type

Primary Psychotherapy Used to Treat Patients with PTSD	Master's-Level Clinicians	Doctoral-Level Psychologists	Psychiatrists/ PNPs
CPG-endorsed psychotherapy			
Cognitive processing therapy***	28.3[a]	39.5[a]	12.4[b]
Exposure therapy or prolonged exposure ***	13.7[a]	31.9[b]	6.9[a]
Eye movement desensitization and reprocessing *	13.6[a]	6.3[a,b]	2.0[b]
Stress inoculation training	0.0	0.0	0.0
Other psychotherapies			
Cognitive behavioral therapy	23.9	13.1	23.6
Supportive counseling***	5.1[a]	0.0[b]	16.6[a]
Motivational interviewing***	1.3[a]	0.0[b]	3.1[a]
Cognitive therapy	1.3	1.4	7.4
Acceptance and commitment therapy ***	0.0[a]	0.0[a]	3.5[b]
Other psychotherapies[a,*]	12.8[a,b]	7.8[a]	24.5[b]

NOTES: n = 404. Values with differing superscripts within rows are significantly different at the $p < 0.05$ level based on post hoc paired comparisons using Wald tests for binary and continuous variables and F statistics for categorical outcomes. Providers responded to a comprehensive list of 30 psychotherapy approaches. The subset of eight shown in the table are those that greater than 3 percent of any provider group endorsed as their "primary mode" of psychotherapy for patients with PTSD or that appear as grade-A treatments in the VA/DoD CPG for posttraumatic stress.

[a] Combines all other primary modes of psychotherapy (behavioral therapy/behavioral activation; brain stimulation; complementary and alternative medicine; couples therapy; dialectical behavioral therapy; existential, experiential/gestalt, and humanistic therapy; hypnosis; imagery rehearsal therapy; integrative/eclectic and interpersonal therapy; problem-solving therapy; psychoanalysis, time-limited psychodynamic, traditional psychodynamic, and reality therapy; and Rogerian, seeking-safety, systems, and other types of therapies).

* $p < 0.05$, *** $p < 0.001$ for omnibus tests.

PTSD psychotherapy approach that is a grade-A technique. The difference between Army and Navy providers was not significant ($p = 0.92$). According to our key informants, both Air Force and Army providers are required to receive training in evidence-based psychotherapies for PTSD, which helps explain why Air Force providers selected these approaches more often than Navy providers. However, given Army training initiatives, it is not clear why Army providers do not differ from Navy providers.

Beyond each provider's primary psychotherapy approach, treatments that providers reported ever using to treat a patient with PTSD may reflect additional skills and capacity acquired by the provider. They may also reflect treatments that a provider uses for some patients but not others or, alternatively, approaches that they are trained to deliver but no longer rely on. These results provide additional information on potential workforce capacity to deliver high-quality care for PTSD.

Figure 4.2 shows that the most common psychotherapies that providers have ever delivered to a patient with PTSD are cognitive behavioral therapy (75.9 percent), cognitive processing therapy (65.5 percent), supportive counseling (48.7 percent), and exposure therapy/pro-

Table 4.2
Primary Psychotherapy Approach for PTSD Among Providers Who Delivered Psychotherapy for PTSD in the Past 30 Days, by Service Branch

Primary Psychotherapy Used to Treat Patients with PTSD	Army	Navy	Air Force
CPG-endorsed psychotherapy			
Cognitive processing therapy**	24.8[a]	35.9[a,b]	46.9[b]
Exposure therapy or prolonged exposure*	18.8[a,b]	12.3[a]	28.1[b]
Eye movement desensitization and reprocessing	11.1	5.9	4.6
Stress inoculation training	0.0	0.0	0.0
Other psychotherapies			
Cognitive behavioral therapy**	21.1[b]	27.1[b]	9.0[a]
Supportive counseling	5.9	3.3	1.7
Motivational interviewing***	1.5[a]	0.6[a]	0.0[b]
Cognitive therapy	2.7	2.3	0.6
Acceptance and commitment therapy***	0.6[a]	0.8[a]	0.0[b]
Other psychotherapies[1]	13.6	11.8	9.1

NOTES: n = 404. Values with differing superscripts within rows are significantly different at the $p < 0.05$ level based on post hoc paired comparisons using Wald tests for binary and continuous variables and F statistics for categorical outcomes. Providers responded to a comprehensive list of 30 psychotherapy approaches. The subset of eight approaches in the table are those that greater 3 percent of any provider group endorsed as their "primary mode" of psychotherapy for patients with PTSD or that appear as grade-A PTSD treatments in the VA/DoD CPG.

[1] Combines all other primary modes of psychotherapy (behavioral therapy/behavioral activation; brain stimulation; complementary and alternative medicine; couples therapy; dialectical behavioral therapy; existential, experiential/gestalt, and humanistic therapy; hypnosis; imagery rehearsal therapy; integrative/eclectic and interpersonal therapy; problem-solving therapy; psychoanalysis, time-limited psychodynamic, traditional psychodynamic, and reality therapy; and Rogerian, seeking-safety, systems, and other types of therapies).

* $p < 0.05$, ** $p < 0.01$, *** $p < 0.001$.

longed exposure (47.8 percent). Approximately two-thirds (69.1 percent) of providers indicated that they had ever used a CPG-endorsed psychotherapy for PTSD (i.e., cognitive processing therapy, exposure therapy/prolonged exposure, eye movement desensitization and reprocessing, or stress inoculation training). As shown in Table 4.3, this number differed significantly across provider types ($p < 0.001$). More than four-fifths of master's-level clinicians (84.6 percent) and doctoral-level psychologists (91.1 percent) indicated that they had delivered at least one CPG-endorsed psychotherapy for PTSD; the groups did not differ significantly from one another ($p = 0.25$). However, both groups were about twice as likely as the subset of psychiatrists/PNPs who provided psychotherapy (36.6 percent of psychiatrists/PNPs) to have delivered a CPG-concordant psychotherapy at least once ($ps < 0.001$). Even for providers who did not identify a CPG-endorsed PTSD psychotherapy as their primary approach for PTSD, there appeared to be a depth of familiarity with these approaches among master's-level clinicians and psychologists. The same was not true for psychiatrists/PNPs, many of whom had never delivered a PTSD psychotherapy that the VA/DoD CPG identifies as "effective."

The percentage of providers who indicated that they had ever delivered at least one of the CPG-endorsed psychotherapies for PTSD was not significantly different across service

Figure 4.2
PTSD Psychotherapy Approaches Ever Used Among Providers Who Delivered Psychotherapy for PTSD in the Past 30 Days

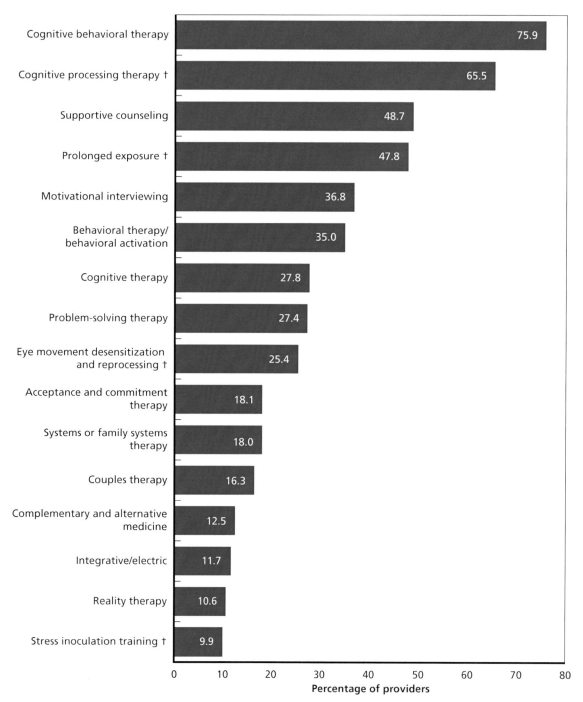

NOTE: † = Psychotherapies identified as recommended treatments for PTSD in the VA/DoD CPG for Post-Traumatic Stress.

RAND RR1692-4.2

Table 4.3
PTSD Psychotherapy Approaches Ever Used Among Providers Who Delivered Psychotherapy for PTSD in the Past 30 Days, by Provider Type

Psychotherapies Ever Used to Treat a Patient with PTSD	Master's-Level Clinicians	Doctoral-Level Psychologists	Psychiatrists/ PNPs
CPG-endorsed psychotherapy			
Cognitive processing therapy***	67.7[a]	77.0[a]	27.9[b]
Exposure therapy or prolonged exposure***	39.9[a]	68.7[b]	18.9[c]
Eye movement desensitization and reprocessing**	34.9[a]	19.8[a,b]	8.3[b]
Stress inoculation training	13.1	9.0	1.5
Other psychotherapies			
Cognitive behavioral therapy***	80.5[a]	78.0[a]	54.7[b]
Supportive counseling**	60.2[a]	31.7[b]	55.3[a]
Motivational interviewing	41.2	33.8	30.3
Behavioral therapy/behavioral activation	29.5[a,b]	45.0[a]	26.9[b]
Cognitive therapy	29.3	25.2	29.4
Problem-solving therapy*	37.4[a]	17.9[b]	19.4[b]
Acceptance and commitment therapy**	11.7[a]	29.6[b]	8.9[a]
Systems or family systems therapy***	29.2[a]	8.8[b]	4.7[b]
Couples therapy*	23.3[a]	9.4[b]	11.1[a,b]
Complementary and alternative medicine (e.g., meditation, acupuncture)	12.4	12.0	14.5
Integrative/eclectic	9.3	14.3	12.3
Reality therapy	15.7[a]	6.6[a,b]	4.4[b]

NOTES: n = 404. Values with differing superscripts within rows are significantly different at the $p < 0.05$ level based on post hoc paired comparisons using Wald tests for binary and continuous variables and F statistics for categorical outcomes. Providers responded to a comprehensive list of 30 psychotherapy approaches. The subset of 16 approaches in the table are those that were endorsed as having been used by at least 10 percent of all providers or that are grade-A treatments in the VA/DoD CPG for posttraumatic stress.

* $p < 0.05$, ** $p < 0.01$, *** $p < 0.001$.

branches ($p = 0.07$; see Table 4.2 for results by specific psychotherapy). The majority of providers working within the Air Force (88.0 percent), Army (79.0 percent), and Navy (76.0 percent) reported that they had experience delivering at least one CPG-endorsed technique.

Because we viewed the items assessing whether a CPG-endorsed technique had ever been delivered as an indirect assessment of potentially untapped workforce capacity to deliver guideline-concordant care, we also examined the results limited to those providers who did not select a CPG-concordant psychotherapy as their primary technique. We wanted to understand whether this group might be able to deliver guideline-concordant psychotherapy even if it were not currently incentivized to do so. Among providers who did not rely on a CPG-concordant PTSD psychotherapy as their primary approach, 65.2 percent of master's-level clinicians and 60.4 percent of psychologists had used one in the past. This fraction was lower among psychiatrists/PNPs who did not select a CPG-concordant PTSD psychotherapy as their primary approach: 19.5 percent.

Delivery of Guideline-Concordant Psychotherapy Techniques for PTSD

To assess whether providers are delivering psychotherapy techniques consistent with CPG-recommended treatments for PTSD, we relied on a self-report measure developed by Wilk and colleagues (2013) to evaluate provider-reported delivery of cognitive processing therapy, prolonged exposure, and eye movement desensitization and reprocessing. After consulting with the developers of each of these psychotherapies, Wilk and colleagues identified four core therapy techniques that defined cognitive processing therapy according to the developers of the therapy, six core prolonged exposure techniques, and three core eye movement desensitization and reprocessing techniques. The survey included items assessing each of these core techniques. The original scale was modified from a yes/no response format for each technique to a Likert scale assessing the frequency of delivery, which ranged from "never" to "always," so that response options were more consistent with the items assessing psychotherapy techniques for depression (described later).

The items from Wilk and colleagues (2013) are relatively newly developed, so there is no established scoring approach, and the items have not yet been validated in terms of whether providers' self-reported delivery of these techniques corresponds to actual practice. In developing a scoring approach for our survey, we considered whether there might be a social desirability bias to endorse most techniques, but we also wanted to ensure that we captured providers' perceived use of the techniques. Therefore, if a provider indicated that he or she had "never" used the technique with his or her most recent PTSD patient, the provider was coded as not delivering the technique. Providers who indicated any other response in relationship to sessions with their most recent patient (i.e., "almost never" and more frequently) were coded as having delivered the technique. Although "almost never" indicates that the patient rarely received the technique, we interpreted this response as indicating that the patient did receive the technique at least one time. We then computed the percentage of providers who indicated that they had delivered all core therapeutic techniques for the psychotherapy to their most recent patient with PTSD. Given that each technique was identified as core or central to the therapy, we coded the provision of *all* techniques as suggesting fidelity to a given psychotherapy.

Before responding to the psychotherapy techniques items, providers were asked to select the most recent adult patient with PTSD with whom they had a psychological counseling visit and to confirm that this patient had been seen within the previous 30 days. Of the 520 total respondents, 378 confirmed that their most recent PTSD psychotherapy patient had been seen within 30 days. Respondents were encouraged to view the patient's electronic chart while responding to these items, though 72.5 percent (weighted; n = 256) indicated that they did not have access to their most recent PTSD patient's chart when completing the survey. Responses from providers who did not review the patient's chart while completing the survey may be subject to increased recall bias.

Given that early sessions may consist largely of assessment and only some of the techniques included in a particular psychotherapy intervention, with other techniques covered in later sessions, we limited our analyses of employed psychotherapy techniques to providers who had delivered at least four sessions of psychotherapy to a patient with PTSD. Of the 378 survey respondents who had seen a patient with PTSD for psychotherapy in the previous 30 days, 315 respondents had met with their most recent patient for at least four sessions. Providers indicated that a large proportion of PTSD patients were also diagnosed with a comorbid psychiatric condition (83.9 percent); comorbidity did not differ by provider type (p = 0.80) or service branch (p = 0.06). Comorbid diagnoses included depressive disorders (45.0 percent), V-code relational problems (39.6 percent),[3] substance use disorders (23.6 percent), anxiety disorders other than PTSD (19.0 percent), personality disorders (12.6 percent), adjustment disorders (12.0 percent), and other psychiatric diagnoses (9.0 percent).

Two-thirds of providers who had recently delivered psychotherapy for PTSD (69.1 percent) indicated that they had delivered all the core elements of cognitive processing therapy to their most recent patient with PTSD, and an additional 16.3 percent indicated that they had delivered all but one of the core elements. Approximately 27.2 percent indicated that they had delivered all the core elements of prolonged exposure, and an additional 27.6 percent had delivered all but one of the core elements. Finally, 30.3 percent had delivered all the core elements of eye movement desensitization and reprocessing, and an additional 60.3 percent had delivered all but one.

It is curious to note that while only 30.3 percent of providers indicated that cognitive processing therapy was their primary treatment approach for PTSD, more than twice that number reported that they had delivered all the core elements of the treatment (69.1 percent). It may be that the items included in the subscales for a specific therapy are shared across multiple treatment types and our survey therefore lacked the specificity to precisely capture those therapists who delivered a given treatment approach. (For example, a cognitive processing therapy item read, "How often did you encourage this patient to write about the meaning of his or her traumatic event as well as beliefs about why the event happened?") Delivery of all core cognitive processing therapy, prolonged exposure, or eye movement desensitization and reprocessing psychotherapy techniques did not differ significantly across the three provider types (p = 0.42–0.78) or across services (p = 0.30–0.42).

When developing their items, Wilk and colleagues surveyed 110 Army behavioral health providers who had recently provided care to a patient with PTSD (Wilk et al., 2013). Our results for Army providers are somewhat inconsistent with their findings. For example, 62.2 percent of Army behavioral health providers in our sample reported delivering all five critical cognitive processing therapy techniques at some point during their patient's treatment, while only 15 percent in the Wilk sample indicated doing so. Rates of endorsement of all prolonged exposure techniques were similar in our sample (23.3 percent) to rates in Wilk et al.'s sample (21 percent). However, Army providers in that sample (47 percent) appeared to be more likely than Army providers in our sample (31.5 percent) to indicate that they delivered all critical eye movement desensitization and reprocessing techniques.

We see a number of possible explanations for these differences. First, there may have been a policy shift between 2010, when Wilk and colleagues administered their survey, and 2016, when our survey was fielded (e.g., perhaps training and support shifted to focus on cognitive processing therapy). Alternatively, methodological differences between the surveys could be responsible for the discrepancies. For example, Wilk and colleagues (2013) included substance abuse counselors (who may be less likely to deliver psychotherapy of any kind), whereas our study did not. Providers in their sample were required to access patient records via their elec-

---

[3]   Problems between or among members of a relational unit (e.g., parent and child, partners) are assigned diagnostic codes that start with "V" in the *Diagnostic and Statistical Manual of Mental Disorders.* In these cases, the target of treatment is the relational problem, and the patient may not have a corresponding PH condition.

tronic charting system and were prompted to select a random patient. This process may have reduced the bias to report socially desirable answers relative to our method, which prompted providers to consider their most recent patient with PTSD and suggested (but did not require) the use of electronic records as a memory aid. Finally, in Wilk et al.'s survey, providers indicated whether they had delivered a given technique with a yes/no response. Our survey prompted providers to indicate whether they had delivered a technique never, almost never, sometimes, usually, almost always, or always. All responses besides "never" were coded as having delivered the technique. Although "yes" and "almost never" are logically equivalent, the threshold a provider used when deciding whether to respond "yes" was likely higher than that used by those responding "almost never," which could explain why Wilk et al.'s survey rates were lower.

Psychotherapy Approaches for MDD

The VA/DoD CPG for MDD identifies three grade-A psychotherapy treatment options as first-line psychotherapies for the treatment of uncomplicated major depression: (1) cognitive behavioral therapy, (2) interpersonal therapy, and (3) problem-solving therapy. Outside of these three therapies, the VA/DoD practice guidelines identify two other grade-A psychotherapies for MDD but limit the recommendation for their use to specific subgroups of patients: behavioral therapy/behavioral activation for inpatients and patients with severe depression, and electroconvulsive therapy for a highly specific subset of patients with severe MDD (e.g., catatonia or other psychotic symptoms). Our analyses focused on the three grade-A psychotherapies recommended as first-line psychotherapies for the treatment of uncomplicated MDD (cognitive behavioral therapy, interpersonal therapy, and problem-solving therapy).

Our provider survey included a comprehensive list of 30 psychotherapies (see Appendix C, item MDD1, for the complete list) that could be used with an MDD patient. We asked respondents to indicate all psychotherapies that they had ever used to treat a patient with MDD and then to select their "primary mode" of treatment for patients with MDD. Embedded in the list were the three strongly recommended psychotherapies for MDD, along with others that are recommended for a subset of patients with MDD and additional psychotherapies that are not recommended for MDD. This section of the survey was limited to respondents who had provided psychotherapy to at least one patient with MDD in the previous 30 days. Of the total 520 respondents, 413 (79.4 percent) indicated that they had done so.

The most frequently endorsed primary psychotherapy approach for the majority of providers was cognitive behavioral therapy (59.9 percent; Figure 4.3). Very few providers selected the other CPG-recommended first-line psychotherapies for MDD as their primary approach: Less than 1 percent of providers selected problem-solving therapy (0.9 percent) or interpersonal therapy (0.7 percent). About three-fifths (61.4 percent) of providers identified a strongly recommended psychotherapy as their primary psychotherapeutic approach for patients with MDD. This differed significantly by provider type ($p < 0.05$). Specifically, master's-level clinicians (66.6 percent) and doctoral-level psychologists (61.9 percent) had a similar likelihood of selecting a strongly recommended psychotherapy for MDD as their primary approach ($p = 0.56$). Both groups were more likely to do so than psychiatrists/PNPs (45.3 percent, $p < 0.05$). As described for PTSD psychotherapies, if we assume that all "supportive counseling" selected by psychiatrists/PNPs is a guideline-appropriate adjunct to medication management, then the rate of MDD guideline concordance for this group would rise from 45.3 percent to 60.7 percent. See Table 4.4 for more detailed results by provider type for various psychotherapy approaches.

Figure 4.3
Primary Psychotherapy Approach for MDD Among Providers Who Delivered Psychotherapy for MDD in the Past 30 Days

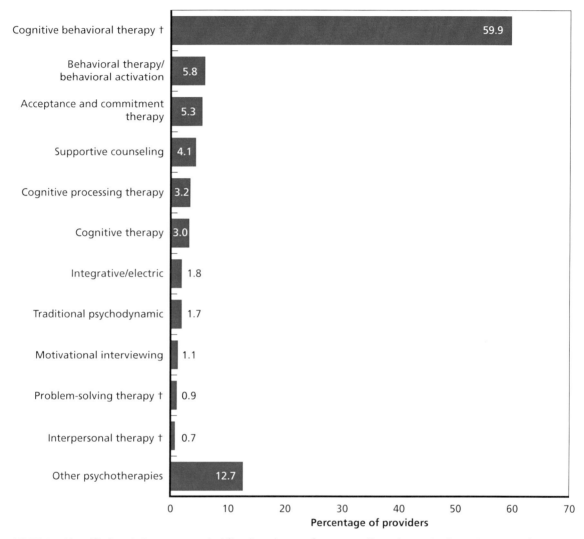

NOTE: † = Identified as CPG-recommended first-line therapy for uncomplicated MDD in the VA/DoD CPG for MDD.
RAND RR1692-4.3

The rate at which providers identified any of the three psychotherapies strongly recommended in the VA/DoD CPG for MDD as their primary approach was not significantly different across service branches ($p = 0.28$). When considering differences for each therapy individually, there were only two significant differences across the service branches (motivational interviewing, $p < 0.001$; interpersonal therapy, $p < 0.001$). These treatments were selected by no more than 2 percent of providers in a given service branch and are not likely to reflect significant training or policy differences across service branches.[4]

---

[4] PH providers who delivered psychotherapy in the Air Force (2.2 percent) and Army (1 percent) were more likely than providers in the Navy (0 percent) to select motivational interviewing as their primary psychotherapy approach for MDD ($p < 0.001$). PH providers who delivered psychotherapy in the Navy (1.3 percent) and Army (0.7 percent) were more likely

Table 4.4
Primary Psychotherapy Approach for MDD Among Providers Who Delivered Psychotherapy for MDD in the Past 30 Days, by Provider Type

Primary Psychotherapy Used to Treat Patients with MDD	Master's-Level Clinicians (%)	Doctoral-Level Psychologists (%)	Psychiatrists/ PNPs (%)
CPG-endorsed psychotherapy			
Cognitive behavioral therapy**	64.8[a]	61.3[a]	41.8[b]
Problem-solving therapy***	1.8[a]	0.0[b]	0.6[a]
Interpersonal therapy***	0.0[a]	0.6[b]	2.9[b]
Other psychotherapies			
Behavioral therapy/behavioral activation	4.0	9.1	2.8
Acceptance and commitment therapy***	0.0[a]	13.3[b]	1.5[c]
Supportive counseling**	3.2[a,b]	0.5[a]	15.5[b]
Cognitive processing therapy	3.4	3.7	1.7
Cognitive therapy	1.7	3.4	5.6
Integrative/eclectic	2.0	0.8	3.6
Traditional psychodynamic***	1.8[a]	0.0[b]	5.4[a]
Motivational interviewing	0.4	0.8	4.0
Other psychotherapies[1]	17.0	6.7	14.6

NOTES: n = 413. Values with differing superscripts within rows are significantly different at the $p < 0.05$ level based on post hoc paired comparisons using Wald tests for binary and continuous variables and F statistics for categorical outcomes. Providers responded to a comprehensive list of 30 psychotherapy approaches. The subset of 11 approaches in the table are those that greater than 3 percent of any provider group endorsed as their "primary mode" of psychotherapy for patients with PTSD or that are recommended as first-line treatment for uncomplicated MDD in the VA/DoD CPG for that condition.

[1] Combines all other primary psychotherapy approaches (brain stimulation, complementary and alternative medicine; couples therapy; dialectical behavioral therapy; existential, experiential/gestalt, exposure therapy or prolonged exposure; eye movement desensitization and reprocessing; humanistic therapy; hypnosis; imagery rehearsal therapy; psychoanalysis; time-limited psychodynamic and reality therapy; and Rogerian, seeking-safety, stress inoculation, systems, and other therapies).

* $p < 0.05$, ** $p < 0.01$, *** $p < 0.001$.

Providers also indicated the psychotherapies that they had ever used to treat a patient with MDD. These additional treatments may be a marker of providers' potential skills and capacity, even if they are not currently relying on the approach. The most common psychotherapies that PH providers had ever delivered to a patient with MDD were cognitive behavioral therapy, followed by supportive counseling and behavioral therapy/behavioral activation (Figure 4.4). Although problem-solving therapy and interpersonal therapy were rarely endorsed as a *primary* treatment approach for MDD (see Figure 4.3), a substantial minority of providers had delivered these first-line, grade-A MDD psychotherapies in the past (28.7 and 15.6 percent, respectively).

than providers in the Air Force (0 percent) to select interpersonal therapy as their primary psychotherapy approach for MDD ($p < 0.001$).

Figure 4.4
MDD Psychotherapy Approaches Ever Used Among Providers Who Delivered Psychotherapy for MDD in the Past 30 Days

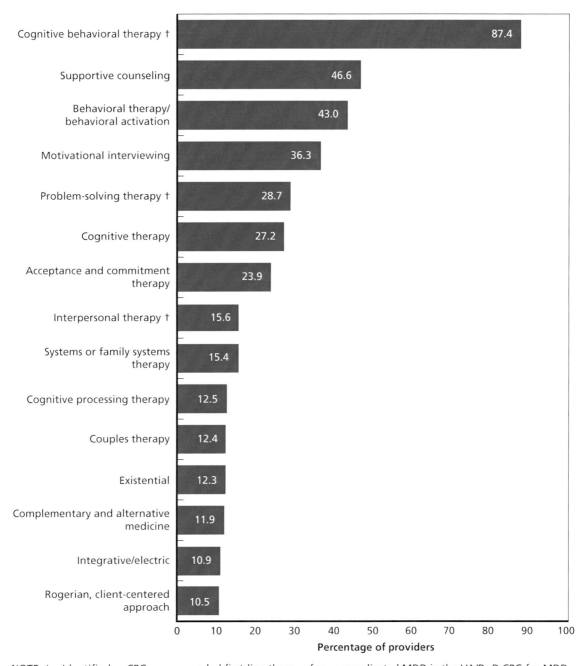

NOTE: † = Identified as CPG-recommended first-line therapy for uncomplicated MDD in the VA/DoD CPG for MDD.
RAND RR1692-4.4

The vast majority of master's-level clinicians (90.1 percent) and doctoral-level psychologists (94.3 percent) indicated that they had delivered at least one first-line, grade-A psychotherapy for MDD, and these provider groups were not significantly different from one another (p = 0.38). However, doctoral-level psychologists were significantly more likely than psychiatrists/PNPs who deliver psychotherapy (78.6 percent) to have ever delivered a strongly recommended psychotherapy for MDD ($p < 0.05$). Despite these differences across provider types, overall a substantial majority of PH providers had delivered a CPG-endorsed first-line, grade-A therapy for MDD, suggesting that a lack of familiarity with these treatments is not a barrier to delivering high-quality care for this condition for most providers.

Table 4.5 compares each type of psychotherapy ever used and shows several statistically significant differences by provider type. In contrast, all comparisons of psychotherapies ever used by service branch were not significant (all $p > 0.05$; not shown).

We also examined the results limited to only those providers who did not select a CPG-concordant psychotherapy as their primary technique for MDD. We wanted to understand whether these providers might be able to deliver guideline-concordant psychotherapy even if they were not currently incentivized to do so. Among master's-level clinicians, 70.4 percent of those who did not select a CPG-concordant psychotherapy as their primary approach for

Table 4.5
MDD Psychotherapy Approaches Ever Used Among Providers Who Delivered Psychotherapy for MDD in the Past 30 Days, by Provider Type

Psychotherapies Ever Used to Treat a Patient with MDD	Master's-Level Clinicians (%)	Doctoral-Level Psychologists (%)	Psychiatrists/ PNPs (%)
CPG-endorsed psychotherapy			
Cognitive behavioral therapy*	87.9[a,b]	92.7[a]	72.9[b]
Problem-solving therapy	33.4	26.2	20.6
Interpersonal therapy	15.0	16.7	14.8
Other psychotherapies			
Supportive counseling*	53.6[a]	33.6[b]	57.4[a]
Behavioral therapy/behavioral activation***	38.7[a,b]	56.8[a]	22.4[b]
Motivational interviewing	40.8	36.1	23.4
Cognitive therapy	26.3	28.9	25.6
Acceptance and commitment therapy***	14.8[a]	42.1[b]	6.8[a]
Systems or family systems therapy**	24.8[a]	8.5[b]	4.3[b]
Cognitive processing therapy	14.9	13.3	3.5
Couples therapy	17.7	7.3	8.6
Existential	4.6	7.3	16.1
Complementary and alternative medicine (e.g., meditation, acupuncture)	11.9	11.6	12.6
Integrative/eclectic	5.9	17.0	11.4
Rogerian, client-centered approach	8.6	15.7	3.5

NOTES: n = 413. Values with differing superscripts within rows are significantly different at the $p < 0.05$ level based on post hoc paired comparisons using Wald tests for binary and continuous variables and F statistics for categorical outcomes. Providers responded to a comprehensive list of 30 psychotherapy approaches. The subset of 11 approaches in the table are those that greater than 3 percent of any provider group endorsed as their "primary mode" of psychotherapy for patients with PTSD or that are recommended as first-line treatment for MDD in the VA/DoD CPG for that condition.

* $p < 0.05$, ** $p < 0.01$, *** $p < 0.001$.

MDD had used one in the past. This rate was 85.0 percent for psychologists and 61.0 percent for psychiatrists/PNPs. Given these percentages, it appears that a sizable percentage of the workforce has some experience delivering guideline-concordant psychotherapies, even though therapists did not currently choose one as their primary approach.

Delivery of Guideline-Concordant Psychotherapy Techniques for MDD

To assess whether providers are delivering psychotherapy techniques consistent with VA/DoD CPG recommendations for MDD, we relied on a measure developed by Hepner and colleagues (2010) to assess provision of cognitive behavioral therapy and interpersonal therapy. Our survey included five items that assessed cognitive behavioral therapy techniques and four items that assessed interpersonal therapy techniques. This measure did not include items assessing problem-solving therapy. Providers indicated the frequency with which they used each technique with their most recent patient on a six-point scale that ranged from "never" to "always." Consistent with the approach used by the measure's developers, we averaged across all techniques associated with cognitive behavioral therapy or interpersonal therapy to create a mean score for each psychotherapy, which we converted to a t-score. Note that this approach differs from the developer-endorsed scoring used for the PTSD items, which was a count of the number of items delivered. We chose to score the items consistent with each developer's recommendations, rather than apply a parallel approach across the two conditions.

Before responding to scale questions, providers were asked to select the most recent adult patient with MDD with whom they had a psychological counseling visit and confirm that this patient had been seen within the previous 30 days. Of the 520 total respondents, 397 confirmed that their most recent MDD psychotherapy patient had been seen within 30 days. Respondents were encouraged to view the patient's electronic chart while responding to the items, though 70.2 percent (weighted; n = 267) indicated that they did not have access to their most recent MDD patient's chart at the time of the survey and instead answered questions about psychotherapy techniques based on their memory of the patient's treatment. Responses from providers who did not review the patient's chart while completing the survey may be subject to increased recall bias.

We limited our analyses of MDD psychotherapy techniques to the 310 providers who had delivered at least four psychotherapy sessions to the identified patient and responded to these items (78.1 percent). Of these patients with MDD, most had other comorbid psychiatric conditions (85.3 percent), which did not differ by provider type ($p = 0.19$) or service branch ($p = 0.12$). Comorbid diagnoses included V-code relational problems (40.8 percent), anxiety disorders other than PTSD (31.2 percent), PTSD (20.2 percent), personality disorders (17.0 percent), substance use disorders (16.8 percent), adjustment disorders (15.6 percent), and other psychiatric diagnoses (6.8 percent).

Nearly all providers who had delivered psychotherapy for MDD indicated that they had delivered all five cognitive behavioral therapy techniques (92.6 percent) and all four interpersonal therapy techniques (96.1 percent). In analyses based on the t-scores for these scales, we found no significant differences by provider type in the delivery of cognitive behavioral therapy ($p = 0.87$) or interpersonal therapy techniques ($p = 0.99$). Service differences were also nonsignificant for both cognitive behavioral therapy ($p = 0.99$) and interpersonal therapy techniques ($p = 0.99$).

Medication Management Within MTFs

Pharmacotherapy for PTSD

We asked all survey respondents to indicate whether they had prescribed a medication or had a medication management visit with an adult patient with PTSD in the previous 30 days. Of the 520 respondents, 186 had provided medication management for PTSD and responded to the subsequent items about their practice (unweighted, 35.8 percent). Providers were asked to select their most recent adult patient with PTSD whom they saw for medication management. They were encouraged to access and refer to the electronic medical record for the patient, though 59.8 percent (weighted; n = 113) indicated that they did not have access to the medical record at the time of the survey. Most of the identified PTSD patients were diagnosed with other comorbid psychiatric conditions (87.9 percent overall), including depressive disorders (49.4 percent), substance use disorders (39.6 percent), V-code relational problems (31.8 percent), anxiety disorders other than PTSD (14.8 percent), personality disorders (13.6 percent), adjustment disorders (11.7 percent), and other psychiatric diagnoses (11.2 percent). We did not explicitly assess other psychiatric or nonpsychiatric disorders. Rates of overall comorbidity did not differ by service branch ($p = 0.96$). Most prescribers indicated that their patient's current prescriptions included psychopharmacologic medication (93.9 percent, weighted; n = 177), and they recorded the patient's current daily, depot (by injection, typically long lasting), and PRN (as-needed) psychopharmacologic medications.[5]

VA/DoD CPG for posttraumatic stress (Management of Post-Traumatic Stress Working Group, 2010) provides a "strong recommendation that clinicians provide" SSRIs and SNRIs to eligible patients with PTSD (grade-A recommendation), noting that the "benefits substantially outweigh harm." Grade-B (i.e., "at least fair evidence of effectiveness") recommendations include mirtazapine, prazosin, tricyclic antidepressants, nefazodone, and monoamine oxidase inhibitors (MAOIs). The CPG also highlights several grade-D drugs for PTSD (i.e., "at least fair evidence that the intervention is ineffective" or that "the harms outweigh the benefits"), with a recommendation "against routinely providing" tiagabine, guanfacine, valproate, topiramate, and risperidone. Finally, benzodiazepines are also identified as ineffective for the treatment of PTSD (grade D), but they are additionally described as harmful in that they could worsen PTSD outcomes. According to the CPG, evidence suggests that "benzodiazepines may actually potentiate the acquisition of fear responses and worsen recovery from trauma" (Management of Post-Traumatic Stress Working Group, 2010). We have reported our findings for benzodiazepines, a grade-D class of drugs that may cause harm, separately from other grade-D drugs that are known to be ineffective for the treatment of PTSD but may not actively worsen outcomes.

When we focused on all psychopharmacologic medication classes, we found the most commonly prescribed classes for providers' most recent patient with PTSD were antidepressants (99.1 percent) and hypnotics (42.4 percent). In the area of guideline-concordant prescribing, nearly 90 percent of prescribers indicated that their most recent PTSD patient was currently prescribed a medication with grade-A evidence to support its effectiveness in treating the condition (Figure 4.5). Although most patients were currently prescribed an effective

---

[5] Providers were not queried about their patient's nonpharmacological medications. Route of administration (e.g., daily or depot) was separated in the survey to allow providers to more easily record their patient's prescriptions. It was not analyzed separately.

Figure 4.5
Grade of Psychopharmacological Medication Prescribed to Most Recent Patient with PTSD Among
Providers Who Delivered a Medication Management Visit for PTSD in the Past 30 Days

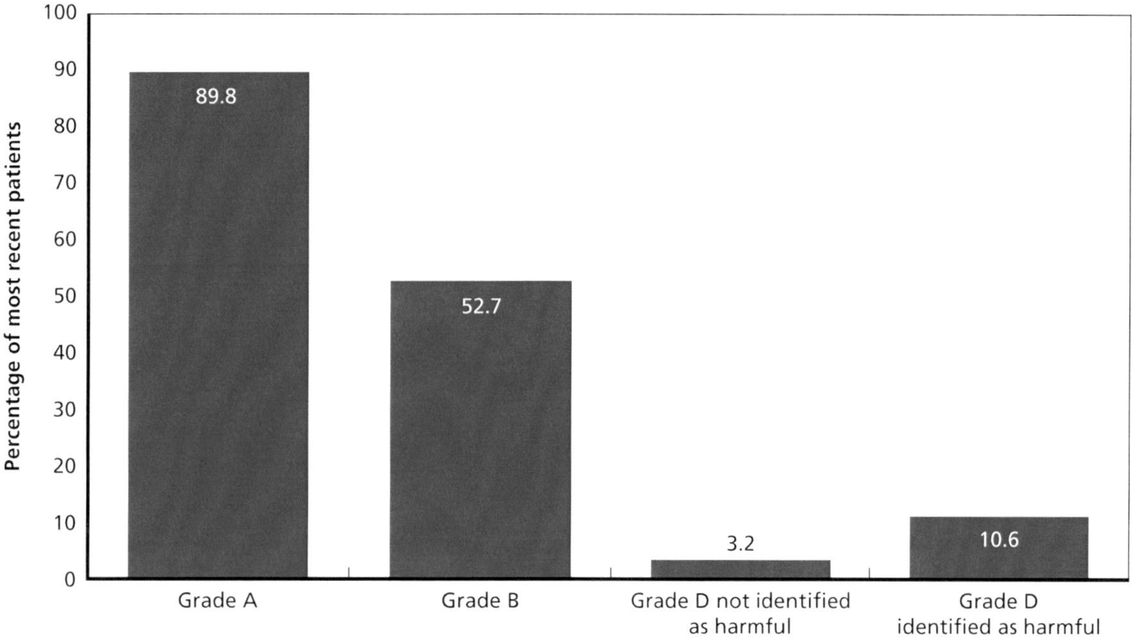

NOTE: n = 177. Grades sum to more than 100 percent because some patients receive multiple medications.
RAND RR1692-4.5

psychopharmacologic treatment for PTSD, one out of ten (10.6 percent) was currently prescribed a medication that the CPG recommend against, given the potential to cause harm and worsen PTSD outcomes. There were no differences across service branches in the proportion of patients receiving grade-A, grade-B, or harmful grade-D medications ($p = 0.39–0.56$). There was a significant service difference in grade-D (not harmful) prescriptions ($p < 0.001$); however, the low rate at which these medications were prescribed made it difficult to interpret the clinical implications.[6]

The majority of prescribers (76.9 percent) indicated that their most recent patient with PTSD was currently prescribed three or fewer prescriptions for psychopharmacological medications (Table 4.6). However, nearly one-quarter of patients were currently prescribed four or more psychopharmacological prescriptions, suggesting that it is important to further investigate prescribing patterns for patients with PTSD. This is consistent with the findings and recommendations of other recent work. For example, a recent review of pharmacy data found that 44.9 percent of service members diagnosed with PTSD received at least four medications over one observation year (Hepner et al., 2017). Differences by service were not significant ($p = 0.55$).

---

[6] Army providers (1.1 percent) were more likely than Air Force (0 percent, $p < 0.001$) and Navy providers (0 percent, $p < 0.001$) to have included a grade-D medication on their most recent PTSD patient's medication list.

Table 4.6
Number of Psychopharmacological Medications Prescribed to Most Recent Patient with PTSD Among Providers Who Delivered a Medication Management Visit for PTSD in the Past 30 Days, by Service Branch

Number of Prescriptions	All Prescribers (%)	Army (%)	Navy (%)	Air Force (%)
1	15.6	11.8	18.8	20.6
2	33.8	34.1	36.9	27.9
3	27.6	21.5	33.8	33.9
4	16.8	24.6	6.8	11.7
5	3.1	5.1	0.0	2.7
6 or more	3.1	2.8	3.8	3.1

NOTE: n = 177.

Pharmacotherapy for MDD

We asked all survey respondents to indicate whether they had prescribed a medication or had a medication management visit with a patient with MDD in the previous 30 days. Of the 520 respondents, 36.2 percent (n = 188) had provided medication management for MDD and responded to the subsequent items about their practice. Providers were asked to select their most recent adult patient with MDD whom they saw for medication management. They were encouraged to access and refer to the patient's electronic medical record, though 63.0 percent (weighted; n = 119) indicated that they did not have access to the medical record at the time of the survey. Most of the identified MDD patients were diagnosed with at least one other comorbid psychiatric condition (81.5 percent overall), including anxiety disorders other than PTSD (33.0 percent), V-code relational problems (24.6 percent), substance use disorders (15.7 percent), PTSD (15.3 percent), adjustment disorders (12.7 percent), personality disorders (9.0 percent), and other psychiatric diagnoses (9.5 percent). Overall rates of comorbidity did not differ by service branch (p = 0.96).

The vast majority of prescribers who had seen a patient with MDD in the previous 30 days for a medication management visit (94.4 percent) indicated that the patient's current prescriptions included psychopharmacologic medication.[7] Each provider then reported the patient's current daily, depot, and PRN psychopharmacologic medications.

According to the VA/DoD CPG for MDD (Management of MDD Working Group, 2009), strongly recommended medications for this condition are SSRIs, SNRIs, bupropion, and mirtazapine. All of these medications are receive a grade-A ranking. The guidelines identify nortriptyline and tricyclic antidepressants as treatments with a grade-B recommendation (i.e., "at lease fair evidence was found that the intervention improves health outcomes and concludes that benefits outweigh harms").

The most commonly prescribed classes of medication for providers' most recent patient with MDD were antidepressants (97.9 percent) and hypnotics (36.1 percent). When considering guideline concordance, 96.9 percent of prescribers indicated that their most recent MDD patient was currently prescribed at least one medication classified as grade A by the VA/DoD CPG for MDD. Only 1 percent were currently prescribed a grade-B medication. There were

---

[7]   Providers were not queried about their patient's nonpharmacological medications.

no significant differences across the service branches with respect to the percentage of MDD patients who were currently prescribed a grade-A medication for MDD ($p = 0.77$); however, there were service branch differences for grade-B prescriptions ($p < 0.001$; Table 4.7).

The majority of prescribers (73.6 percent) indicated that their most recent patient with MDD was currently prescribed two or fewer psychopharmacological medications (Table 4.8). Differences by service were not significant ($p = 0.78$). These findings are somewhat inconsistent with the findings of other recent work. For example, a recent review of pharmacy data found that 31.5 percent of patients with depression received at least four medications over one observation year (Hepner et al., 2017), whereas our provider-reported data showed that 11.6 percent were currently prescribed four or more medications. This discrepancy may be due to a difference in measurement. The current study relies on a self-reported snapshot of a patient's current medications, whereas the Hepner and colleagues study was based on pharmacy data of all psychopharmacological medications prescribed over a year. These differences in methodology should be expected to reveal smaller numbers for the snapshot method and larger numbers in the one-year method.

Table 4.7
Percentage of Providers Who Indicated That Their Most Recent Patient with MDD Was Prescribed a Grade-A or Grade-B Medication for MDD Among Providers Who Delivered a Medication Management Visit for MDD in the Past 30 Days, by Service Branch

Prescription Type	Army	Navy	Air Force
Grade A	97.8	97.0	93.8
Grade B***	0.0[a]	3.1[b]	0.0[a]

NOTES: n = 178. Values with differing superscripts within rows are significantly different at the $p < 0.05$ level based on post hoc paired comparisons using Wald tests. Limited to providers who had delivered a medication management visit for MDD in the past 30 days.

*** $p < 0.001$.

Table 4.8
Number of Psychotropic Medications Prescribed to Providers' Most Recent Patient with MDD, by Service Branch

Number of Prescriptions	All Prescribers (%)	Army (%)	Navy (%)	Air Force (%)
1	31.6	33.9	28.6	29.6
2	42.0	39.9	50.9	31.1
3	14.9	14.1	12.3	22.7
4	9.2	10.8	4.6	13.2
5	0.9	0.0	1.2	3.5
6	1.5	1.3	2.5	0.0

NOTES: n = 178. No providers indicated that their most recent MDD patient was prescribed more than six psychopharmacological medications. Limited to providers who had delivered a medication management visit for MDD in the past 30 days.

Use of Measurement-Based Care

Among the core components of measurement-based care are screening and monitoring patient symptoms with validated instruments (Morris and Trivedi, 2011; Scott and Lewis, 2015). These assessments generate information that can inform treatment planning and adjustments. Providers responded to three questions about the frequency with which they relied on measurement-based care practices using a five-point Likert scale that ranged from "never" to "always." A high proportion of survey respondents indicated that either they or their support staff always screened for PTSD (70.7 percent) and MDD (79.1 percent) with a validated screening instrument. Fewer providers (57.9 percent) indicated that they always use a validated instrument of patient symptoms to inform treatment plan adjustments. There were no significant differences in the rate at which different provider types indicated that they relied on measurement-based care ($p = 0.16–0.51$).[8]

Use of measurement-based care varied significantly across service branches (Figure 4.6). Army providers were significantly more likely than Air Force providers to screen new patients for PTSD with a validated screening instrument ($p < 0.05$). However, this pattern was reversed for MDD, with Air Force providers more likely than both Army and Navy providers to report screening for MDD with a validated instrument ($p < 0.01$). Finally, Air Force providers (63.1 percent) were more likely than Navy providers to use a validated patient symptom scale to update their treatment plans ($p < 0.05$).

Figure 4.6
Practices Consistent with Measurement-Based Care, by Service Branch

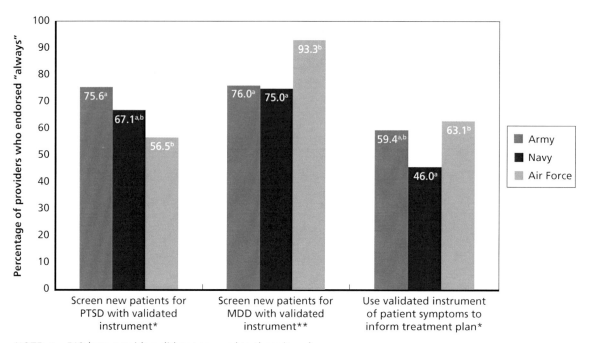

NOTE: n = 518 (two providers did not respond to these items).
* $p < 0.05$, ** $p < 0.01$. Values with differing superscripts within column clusters are significantly different at the $p < 0.05$ level based on post hoc paired comparisons using Wald tests. All respondents had delivered care to a patient with PTSD or MDD in the past 30 days.
RAND *RR1692-4.6*

---

[8]   Other components, such as care management, follow-up, and treatment adjustment, were not measured.

Summary

A similar proportion of MTF psychotherapy providers (about three-fifths) selected a grade-A treatment as their primary psychotherapy approach for both PTSD patients and MDD patients. This reported use of evidence-based treatments suggests some success in promoting evidence-based care, hiring practices to support evidence-based care, and training to improve the delivery of evidence-based care. Among providers who indicated that their primary psychotherapy approach was not a CPG-identified grade-A treatment, a substantial proportion reported delivering a guideline-concordant psychotherapy in the past. This may suggest that there is latent capacity in the workforce that could be tapped, given the right incentives. Approximately 60–85 percent of psychologists and master's-level clinicians who did *not* use a CPG-endorsed psychotherapy as their primary approach to PTSD or MDD had used one in the past. For psychiatrists/PNPs who delivered psychotherapy but did not choose a CPG-endorsed psychotherapy as their primary approach, about three-fifths had experience delivering a CPG-endorsed psychotherapy for MDD in the past, but only one-fifth had experience delivering a CPG-endorsed psychotherapy for PTSD.

Among providers who prescribed and managed psychopharmacological treatments, nine out of ten indicated that their most recent PTSD or MDD patient was currently prescribed a CPG-endorsed, grade-A medication. However, for PTSD medication management, there is room for improvement in terms of prescriptions identified as harmful by the VA/DoD CPG for posttraumatic stress. One-tenth of the medication providers indicated that they were currently prescribing a benzodiazepine to their most recent PTSD patient. Moreover, one-quarter of prescribers indicated that their most recent PTSD patient was currently prescribed four or more medications. This suggests that patients may be receiving a complex mix of medications; a better understanding of the appropriateness of these prescribing patterns would be useful. It is important to note that the survey data did not allow us to assess the extent to which patients were responding well (or poorly) to their current medications and dosages or whether they experienced any side effects.

Psychiatrists/PNPs who delivered psychotherapy were less likely to indicate that they were providing a grade-A psychotherapy for PTSD or MDD when compared with psychologists and master's-level clinicians. Specifically, one out of five psychiatrists/PNPs who delivered psychotherapy chose a CPG-endorsed psychotherapy as his or her primary psychotherapy approach for PTSD patients, and less than half chose a CPG-endorsed MDD psychotherapy. There are several possible explanations for these results. First, psychiatrists/PNPs often endorsed supportive therapy as their primary approach (16.6 percent for PTSD; 15.5 percent for MDD), which is an adjunct to medication management. Therefore, if these patients received guideline-concordant medication treatment, then supportive therapy might be a clinical management strategy to encourage treatment compliance and address patient concerns regarding the medication treatment. Our survey data also suggest that some psychiatrists/PNPs may be using non–guideline-concordant psychotherapies for PTSD, in particular. For example, one-quarter (24.5 percent) selected "other" psychotherapies as their primary PTSD psychotherapy approach (a combined category that excluded grade-A psychotherapies and supportive counseling but that included nonvalidated PTSD treatments, such as psychodynamic therapy, acceptance and commitment therapy, and motivation interviewing). These patterns of reported psychotherapy use suggest both key strengths and potential areas for improvement.

About three-quarters of survey respondents indicated that either they or their support staff always screened for PTSD and MDD with a validated screening instrument. However, fewer providers indicated that they always use a validated instrument of patient symptoms to inform treatment plan adjustments. There were no significant differences in the rate at which different provider types indicated that they relied on measurement-based care, and service branch differences were inconsistent across disorders.

CHAPTER FIVE

Facilitators and Barriers to Provision of Guideline-Concordant Care for PTSD and MDD

In this chapter, using data from our provider survey and key informant discussions, we examine several factors that may affect the degree to which MTF providers deliver guideline-concordant care for PTSD and MDD. We first focus on the survey data on potential facilitators to providing guideline-concordant care, including training, supervision, and confidence in delivering guideline-concordant care. Then, we address potential barriers, including characteristics of providers' practices, such as the number and timing of visits, structural and organizational barriers, and providers' perceived confidence in delivering these treatments, incorporating both provider survey data and context from our key informant discussions.

Training and Supervision in Guideline-Concordant Psychotherapies

Several institutions are integral to training the MHS PH workforce. The Uniformed Services University of Health Sciences (USU) trains doctors, nurses, and public health professionals for use in both domestic and foreign territories (Uniformed Services University, 2016). The Center for Deployment Psychology, a component of the USU established as part of a VA/DoD interagency effort, provides trainings and workshops for PH providers across the MHS. Trainings are often centered on frequently encountered PH conditions (e.g., PTSD and MDD), and two-to-three-day workshops provide opportunities for providers to learn evidence-based psychotherapies, including cognitive behavioral therapy for MDD, as well as prolonged exposure and cognitive processing therapy for PTSD. Providers who complete these trainings are eligible for continuing education credits but do not receive certification in these treatment approaches. Furthermore, DCoE offers multiple resources and training opportunities on delivery of high-quality, evidence-based care for various PH conditions, including PTSD and MDD (Defense Centers of Excellence for Psychological Health & Traumatic Brain Injury, 2016).

Although DHA promotes training in evidence-based psychotherapy, primary responsibility for identifying and addressing providers' training needs rests with the service branches, which also determine which training platforms and instructors will be used. Some service branches offer additional training opportunities for their PH providers. According to our key informants, the Army requires all PH providers to complete training in evidence-based psychotherapies (e.g., prolonged exposure and cognitive processing therapy for PTSD) and has multiple mechanisms for providing this training, including the U.S. Army Medical Department Center and School. The Air Force requires that all PH providers receive training in prolonged exposure through the Center for Deployment Psychology. To our knowledge, the Navy does not require or provide specific training on evidence-based psychotherapies.

Given that training in these approaches is a critical facilitator in ensuring the use of evidence-based techniques, we explored the extent to which providers reported receiving training and supervision in a variety of evidence-based interventions. In the following sections, we describe the findings from our survey analyses.

Provider Survey Responses

We sought to identify providers who had received at least a minimum amount of training and supervision in each grade-A PTSD and MDD psychotherapy, as this experience may allow them to deliver the psychotherapy competently. Identifying the proportion of the workforce with this training can provide insight into untapped capacity and potential to deliver CPG-concordant care for PTSD and MDD within MTFs. To identify the proportion of providers who may have this capacity, we defined *minimally adequate training/supervision* as having received more than eight hours of training and at least one hour of supervision in a given modality. To ensure that we measured capacity only among providers who delivered psychotherapy, we limited our analyses of training/supervision to those who reported doing so in the previous 30 days.

Figure 5.1 shows the percentage of providers who had minimally adequate levels of training to deliver each VA/DoD CPG-identified grade-A psychotherapy for PTSD and each psychotherapy for MDD recommended by the CPG as a first-line treatment for uncomplicated major depression.

Figure 5.1
Percentage with Minimally Adequate Training/Supervision in Psychotherapies for PTSD and MDD Among Providers Who Delivered Psychotherapy for PTSD or MDD in the Past 30 Days

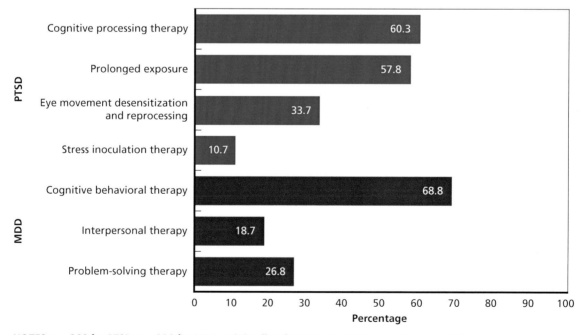

NOTES: n = 366 for PTSD; n = 386 for MDD. Minimally adequate training/supervision was defined as more than eight hours of training and at least one hour of supervision in a given modality.
RAND *RR1692-5.1*

Among providers who had delivered any psychotherapy in the previous 30 days, 76.5 percent indicated that they had received minimally adequate training/supervision in at least one grade-A PTSD psychotherapy, and 69.2 percent indicated that they had received minimally adequate training/supervision in at least one first-line MDD psychotherapy. Approximately three-fifths (59.2 percent) indicated they had received minimally adequate training/supervision in both a grade-A PTSD psychotherapy and a first-line MDD psychotherapy. Analyses of these composite variables revealed there were significant differences across provider types with respect to the proportion of respondents who had received minimally adequate training in at least one grade-A psychotherapy for PTSD ($p < 0.001$) or MDD ($p < 0.01$). For PTSD psychotherapies, the proportions of psychologists (83.6 percent) and master's-level clinicians (77.9 percent) with this training were not significantly different ($p = 0.55$), but both provider types were significantly more likely than psychiatrists/PNPs (52.4 percent) to have received minimally adequate training/supervision ($p < 0.01$). For minimally adequate training/supervision in a first-line MDD psychotherapy, psychologists (83.0 percent) and psychiatrists/PNPs (73.4 percent) did not differ significantly, but both groups were more likely than master's-level clinicians (56.0 percent, $p < 0.05$) to have received minimal training/supervision. Table 5.1 summarizes provider differences in training/supervision for each of the CPG-endorsed psychotherapies for PTSD and MDD.

When we analyzed service differences in the proportion of providers who had received minimally adequate training in at least one grade-A psychotherapy for PTSD ($p = 0.66$) or MDD ($p = 0.74$), there were no significant differences. However, when we examined specific psychotherapies, there were differences only for prolonged exposure ($p < 0.001$) and eye movement desensitization and reprocessing ($p < 0.001$). For prolonged exposure, Air Force providers (66.9 percent) and Army providers (58.3 percent) were significantly more likely than Navy pro-

Table 5.1
Percentage with Minimally Adequate Training/Supervision in Psychotherapies for PTSD and MDD Among Providers Who Delivered PTSD or MDD Psychotherapy in the Past 30 Days, by Provider Type

Treatment	Master's-Level Clinicians	Doctoral-Level Psychologists	Psychiatrists/ PNPs
Evidence-based PTSD psychotherapies			
Cognitive processing therapy**	60.6[a]	67.2[a]	40.5[b]
Prolonged exposure***	53.5[a]	70.7[b]	36.2[c]
Eye movement desensitization and reprocessing***	42.5[a]	31.9[a]	9.7[b]
Stress inoculation training	9.2	14.2	6.3
Evidence-based MDD psychotherapies			
Cognitive behavioral therapy**	56.0[a]	82.2[b]	73.3[b]
Interpersonal therapy***	7.4[a]	22.2[b]	42.6[c]
Problem-solving therapy	20.9	31.6	32.1

**$p < 0.01$, ***$p < 0.001$.

NOTES: n = 366 for PTSD; n = 386 for MDD. Values with differing superscripts within rows are significantly different at the $p < 0.05$ level based on post hoc paired comparisons using Wald tests. Minimally adequate training/supervision was defined as more than eight hours of training and at least one hour of supervision in a given modality.

viders (43.0 percent) to have received minimally adequate training/supervision in prolonged exposure ($p < 0.05$). For eye movement desensitization and reprocessing, Army providers (41.5 percent) were two to three times more likely than Air Force (11.9 percent) and Navy providers (22.9 percent) to have received training/supervision ($p < 0.001$). These findings are consistent with efforts by the Air Force to require training in prolonged exposure for all PH providers and Army requirements that PH providers receive training in multiple evidence-based psychotherapies. To our knowledge, the Navy does not have an evidence-based psychotherapy training requirement.

We also assessed the degree to which respondents felt confident delivering the identified grade-A treatments for PTSD and MDD. Figure 5.2 and Table 5.2 show the percentage of providers who indicated that they were "very confident" in their ability to deliver each treatment approach. For medication management, the data are limited to only those providers who indicated that they had a medication management visit with a PTSD or MDD patient in the previous 30 days. For psychotherapy, the data are limited to only those providers who indicated that they had delivered psychotherapy to a patient with PTSD or MDD in the previous 30 days.

Figure 5.2
Percentage of Providers Who Were "Very Confident" in Their Ability to Deliver Treatment for PTSD and MDD Among Providers Who Delivered PTSD or MDD Services in the Past 30 Days

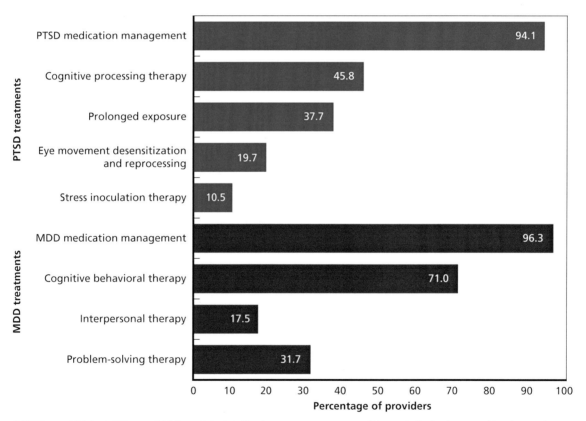

NOTES: n = 366 for PTSD; n = 386 for MDD. Medication management confidence is limited to psychiatrists and psychiatric nurse practitioners who delivered a medication management visit in the previous 30 days. Psychotherapy confidence is limited to providers who delivered a psychotherapy visit in the previous 30 days.
RAND RR1692-5.2

Table 5.2
Percentage of Providers Who Were "Very Confident" in Their Ability to Deliver Treatment for PTSD and MDD Among Providers Who Delivered PTSD or MDD Services in the Past 30 Days, by Provider Type

Treatment	Master's-Level Clinicians	Doctoral-Level Psychologists	Psychiatrists/ PNPs
Evidence-based PTSD treatment			
Medication management[1]	NA	NA	93.4
Cognitive processing therapy[2],***	44.7[a]	52.6[a]	14.6[b]
Prolonged exposure[2],***	27.3[a]	50.9[b]	12.6[c]
Eye movement desensitization and reprocessing[2],**	25.0[a]	15.1[a]	1.9[b]
Stress inoculation training[2],*	10.5[a]	11.0[a]	1.5[b]
Evidence-based MDD treatment			
Medication management[1]	NA	NA	95.7
Cognitive behavioral therapy[2],***	58.9[a]	87.5[b]	48.4[a]
Interpersonal therapy[2]	15.6	15.1	25.7
Problem-solving therapy[2]	33.3	28.4	24.4

NOTES: Values with differing superscripts within rows are significantly different at the $p < 0.05$ level based on post hoc paired comparisons using Wald tests. Due to missing values, the number of responses on each item varied. PTSD (n = 393) numbers ranged from 391 to 392; MDD (n = 409) numbers ranged from 407 to 408.

* $p < 0.05$, ** $p < 0.01$, *** $p < 0.001$.

[1] Limited to psychiatrists and psychiatric nurse practitioners who reported a medication management visit in the previous 30 days. This excludes a small number of psychologists who were licensed to prescribe medications.

[2] Limited to providers who reported a psychotherapy visit for the given condition in the previous 30 days.

Almost all psychiatrists/PNPs were "very confident" in their ability to deliver medication management for PTSD and MDD (see Figure 5.2). This high confidence seems to map well to the provision of high-quality, evidence-based care as described in Chapter Four (see section titled Medication Management Within MTFs). Psychotherapy providers were far less confident in their ability to deliver grade-A PTSD psychotherapies. Fewer than half of providers (45.8 percent) felt very confident in their ability to deliver cognitive processing therapy, and this was the PTSD psychotherapy with the highest provider confidence level. Of the grade-A psychotherapies identified as first-line therapies for uncomplicated MDD, a large cohort of providers (71 percent) felt very confident in their ability to deliver cognitive behavioral therapy, but there was less confidence for interpersonal therapy and problem-solving therapy. For each psychotherapy measured, minimally adequate training in each psychotherapy was positively associated with self-reported confidence delivering that psychotherapy ($ps < 0.05$).

Master's-level clinicians and doctoral-level psychologists tend to have caseloads with a strong focus on delivery of psychotherapy, whereas psychiatrists/PNPs typically spend less time delivering psychotherapy and more time managing medication. Given this difference in clinical responsibilities, it is not surprising that master's-level clinicians and psychologists were more confident than psychiatrists/PNPs in their ability to deliver all grade-A PTSD psychotherapies (Table 5.2). For the grade-A, first-line MDD psychotherapies, this general pattern did not hold. Psychiatrists/PNPs did not differ significantly from other providers in their confidence in delivering interpersonal therapy or problem-solving therapy. Finally, confidence in delivering cognitive behavioral therapy for MDD was highest for psychologists and lower for psychiatrists/PNPs and master's-level clinicians (who did not differ significantly from one another).

The only item for which there was a significant service difference was confidence in delivery of eye movement desensitization and reprocessing for PTSD ($p < 0.01$). Army providers (25.7 percent) were more likely to indicate that they were "very confident" in their ability to deliver eye movement desensitization and reprocessing than were Air Force (4.0 percent, $p < 0.01$) and Navy providers (9.9 percent, $p < 0.05$). Air Force and Navy providers did not differ significantly ($p = 0.27$).

Perceived Barriers to Delivering Guideline-Concordant Treatment

Barriers to the implementation of high-quality PH care may exist at several levels. To understand the nature, type, and prevalence of these barriers, we drew on both our key informant discussions and our provider survey. While survey results highlighted barriers to high-quality PH care from providers' perspectives, we gleaned additional insights on challenges from the key informant discussions. The perspectives of these individuals provide higher-level insight into issues associated with military culture and the environment in which providers practice, which may affect whether and how providers can actually deliver high-quality care. In the discussion that follows, we have grouped barriers to the implementation of evidence-based care, as cited by our key informants, into patient factors and structural/organizational factors.

Patient Factors

Key informants mentioned several patient factors that can preclude delivery of high-quality PH care. For example, many noted that the stigma surrounding PH issues remains a barrier to accessing treatment for service members, despite service-level and DoD-wide efforts to change this perception. This is consistent with findings from prior published literature (Acosta et al., 2014). Furthermore, increased operational tempo and personnel tempo, which assess the intensity of military activity via equipment usage and the amount of time service members spend away from their home base, respectively (Levy et al., 2001), can make it difficult for patients to adhere to regular appointment schedules and thus may preclude a service member from completing a full course of treatment. For example, prolonged exposure therapy requires patients to attend between nine and twelve 90-minute sessions (Powers et al., 2010), a potentially challenging time commitment. Another recent study found that patients reported difficulty getting follow-up appointments and noted concern over provider turnover (Tanielian et al., 2016). These factors may also serve as barriers to patients receiving high-quality care.

Structural and Organizational Factors

Key informants noted that the fragmented or disconnected nature of PH systems, both across and within branches of service, negatively affects providers' ability to deliver high-quality care. Within a service branch, inconsistent communication between MTF providers and other regional personnel, a lack of tools for information sharing across providers or locations, and a dearth of care coordination within and between direct and purchased care providers were all mentioned as features of military PH systems that prevent the delivery of high-quality PH care. Of note, no key informants from the Army identified these issues as barriers to delivering high-quality PH care, presumably because the Army's restructured PH systems have increased communication and integration between multiple key stakeholders.

Provider Perceptions of Barriers

Our key informant discussions provided insights into some system- and organizational-level issues that may affect individual provider behavior, but we also asked providers to respond to a series of 26 survey items that assessed potential barriers to delivering guideline-concordant care for PTSD and MDD. Providers responded to each statement by selecting "strongly disagree," "disagree," "neither disagree nor agree," "agree," or "strongly agree." Table 5.3 shows items for which more than 15 percent of providers selected "strongly agree" (or "strongly disagree," if the item was reverse-coded). We focused on strong agreement or disagreement as an indicator that the item strongly resonated with the provider's experience. The top two barriers were related to support for professional training. About 30 percent of providers strongly agreed that limitations on travel prevented them from obtaining additional clinical training. A similar proportion of providers strongly agreed that their schedule lacked the protected time necessary to attend workshops or seminars to improve their clinical skills. Although many providers have received minimally adequate training in evidence-based therapies, barriers to receiving training may make it difficult for those without training in specific modalities to catch up and for those with limited training to reach competence. Providers also identified structural barriers associated with MTF- or MHS-level resources. Specifically, they indicated that their clinical schedules did not allow them to see their patients as frequently as they would like and that they lacked support from case managers. About 18 percent of providers strongly agreed that patients' military duties (e.g., a permanent change of station or deployment) limited the provider's ability to deliver high-quality care. Finally, one-quarter of providers strongly agreed that nonspecific elements of therapy, such as good rapport or empathy, were largely responsible for treatment success. When a provider believes that these general aspects of therapy explain

Table 5.3
Top Barriers to Delivery of Guideline-Concordant Care Among Providers Who Delivered Services for PTSD or MDD in the Past 30 Days

Response	% of Providers Who Strongly Agree/Strongly Disagree[a]
Limitations on travel prevent me from receiving additional training.	31.7
I have protected time in my schedule to attend workshops/seminars to improve my clinical skills. (reverse-scored)	28.6
Nonspecific aspects of therapy, like good rapport, are the best predictors of treatment success.	25.7
I don't have the time in my schedule to see patients as often as I would like.	24.7
My patients' military duties limit their ability to receive appropriate care (e.g., patient PCS, deployment, irregular work schedules).	17.6
I am well supported by case managers (e.g., coordinating interdisciplinary care, follow-up with patients who do not attend appointments). (reverse-scored)	17.4

NOTES: n = 503. Due to missing values, number of responses for each item ranges from 498 to 503.
[a] Some items were reverse-scored.

success, he or she may be less motivated to deliver specific evidence-based treatments with high fidelity. The rate of endorsement for each of the top six barriers did not differ by provider type (p = 0.08–0.64) or by service branch (p = 0.08–0.84). Other, less commonly endorsed barriers included negative attitudes toward standardized practice, provider burnout, and concerns that CPGs interfere with patient-centered care (see Appendix C, items B1–B26, for complete list of barriers).

Practice Patterns That Affect the Delivery of CPG-Recommended Care

Most evidence-based psychotherapies have manuals specifying the minimum number of sessions that should be delivered and the frequency with which therapists should see their patients. If MTF therapists' schedules are constrained in such a way that they cannot see patients as often or as frequently as recommended in treatment manuals, it may have a negative impact on the quality of care that they are able to provide. To assess this possible barrier, we asked survey respondents to estimate the average number of visits they completed with a patient with PTSD in a typical course of treatment. In addition, respondents were asked how often they were able to see a patient with PTSD, taking into account their current caseload. They were then asked to report on these practice patterns for patients with MDD.

Figure 5.3 shows the distribution of the typical number of psychotherapy or medication management visits for PTSD and MDD. More than 80 percent of respondents reported that they typically saw both PTSD and MDD patients for eight or more sessions (84 percent for PTSD; 83 percent for MDD). Providers were more likely to report completing 12 or more visits with PTSD patients (48.6 percent) than MDD patients (35.8 percent; p < 0.001). While patients with PTSD or MDD may vary in terms of the total number of psychotherapy sessions needed to achieve response or remission, it has been suggested that eight sessions may be the minimum number for delivery of an evidence-based psychotherapy (Shin et al., 2014). These results suggest that providers are typically able to see patients with PTSD or MDD for

Figure 5.3
Typical Number of Visits with PTSD and MDD Patients Among Providers Who Delivered Services for PTSD or MDD in the Past 30 Days

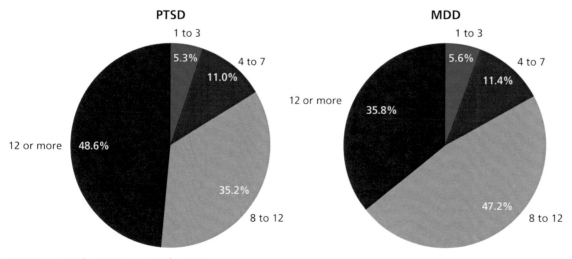

NOTE: n = 507 for PTSD; n = 510 for MDD.
RAND RR1692-5.3

enough sessions to provide at least a minimal dose. There were no significant differences across provider types or across the services in the number of sessions providers were able to deliver to their patients with PTSD or MDD (p = 0.09–0.87).

Given the difference in practice patterns between providers who focused on medication management and those who focused on psychotherapy, we ran secondary analyses that excluded providers who indicated that they had delivered both medication management and psychotherapy in the previous 30 days. The average duration of PTSD treatment among providers who delivered medication management only was not significantly different from the average duration reported by providers who delivered psychotherapy only (p = 0.31). However, for MDD patients, psychotherapy-only providers (39.2 percent) were more likely than medication management–only providers (17.0 percent) to report seeing their patients for 12 or more sessions (p < 0.001).

Although the number of sessions in a typical course of treatment is an important indicator of whether providers can deliver an evidence-based psychotherapy, it is also important that providers are able to see patients at regular intervals that support ongoing clinical progress (Erekson, Lambert, and Eggett, 2015). Evidence-based psychotherapies were typically delivered in weekly sessions when they were evaluated in efficacy trials (Nacasch et al., 2011), though biweekly or monthly sessions can be used when patients are nearing the end of their course of treatment (i.e., tapering of sessions). Medication management visits are more typically scheduled monthly and then less often after the patient is stable. Approximately 40 percent of providers reported that they typically saw patients with PTSD or MDD at least weekly (Figure 5.4). Overall, they reported seeing PTSD patients more frequently than MDD patients

Figure 5.4
Frequency of Visits with PTSD and MDD Patients Among Providers Who Delivered Services for PTSD or MDD in the Past 30 Days

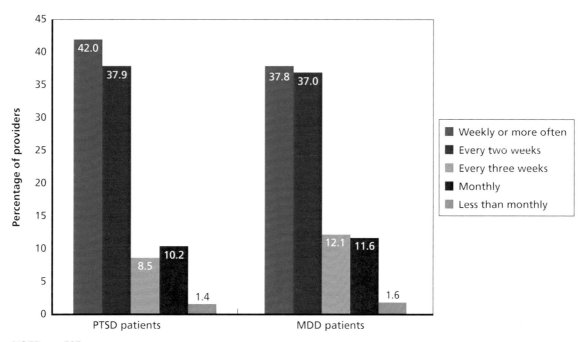

NOTE: n = 507.

($p < 0.001$). Notably, one-fifth of providers reported seeing PTSD patients every three weeks or less often, while a quarter of providers reported doing so for MDD patients. Patients seen with this frequency may have more difficulty receiving the benefit of an evidence-based psychotherapy (Reardon et al., 2002).

Providers may vary in the frequency with which they typically see patients. Specifically, psychiatrists/PNPs are more likely to conduct medication management than psychotherapy, which is more likely to be associated with monthly visits. As expected, psychiatrists/PNPs reported that they saw PTSD and MDD patients less often (modal response of "monthly") than did master's-level clinicians and psychologists (Table 5.4). More than 85 percent of master's-level clinicians and psychologists reported that they saw their patients with PTSD or MDD either weekly or every other week. However, fewer than half of these providers reported seeing patients weekly, a frequency that may be more conducive to ongoing psychotherapy. The exception was that just over half of master's-level clinicians were able to see PTSD patients weekly.

Because some psychiatrists/PNPs deliver both medication management and psychotherapy, to clarify the results, we ran a sensitivity analysis to assess session frequency among providers who deliver medication management and do not deliver psychotherapy, relative to providers who deliver psychotherapy and do not deliver medication management. As expected, the frequency with which medication management–only providers saw their MDD and PTSD patients was lower than among psychotherapy-only providers ($p < 0.001$). Among psychotherapy-only providers, 45 percent saw their PTSD patients weekly or more often, 42 percent saw their PTSD patients every two weeks, 10 percent saw their PTSD patients every three weeks, and 4 percent of providers saw their PTSD patients less than once a month. A similar pattern held for psycho-

Table 5.4
Frequency of Visits with PTSD and MDD Patients Among Providers Who Delivered Services for PTSD or MDD in the Past 30 Days, by Provider Type

Visit Frequency	Master's-Level Clinicians	Doctoral-Level Psychologists	Psychiatrists/PNPs
PTSD patients (%) (n = 507)***	a	a	b
Weekly or more often	52.8	42.8	17.9
Every two weeks	35.0	47.1	28.7
Every three weeks	6.4	8.4	13.3
Monthly	5.1	1.3	35.7
Less than monthly	0.7	0.4	4.5
MDD patients (%) (n = 510)***	a	a	b
Weekly or more often	44.6	43.8	13.4
Every two weeks	41.7	41.2	20.1
Every three weeks	8.1	13.1	18.8
Monthly	5.2	1.5	42.0
Less than monthly	0.4	0.4	5.8

NOTES: n = 519. Values with differing superscripts within rows are significantly different at the $p < 0.05$ level based on post hoc paired comparisons using F statistics.
**$p < 0.01$, ***$p < 0.001$.

therapy-only providers and their MDD patients. Of these providers, 49 percent saw their MDD patients weekly or more often, 41 percent saw their MDD patients every two weeks, 7 percent saw their MDD patients every three weeks, and 4 percent of providers saw their MDD patients monthly or less frequently. Medication management–only providers saw patients comparatively less frequently. Among these providers, 17 percent, 21 percent, and 14 percent saw their PTSD patients weekly or more often, every two weeks, or every three weeks (respectively), and 48 percent of medication management–only providers saw their patients monthly or less. Furthermore, 19 percent, 29 percent, and 9 percent of medication management–only providers saw their MDD patients weekly or more often, every two weeks, or every three weeks (respectively), and 43 percent of these providers saw their MDD patients monthly or less frequently.

The frequency with which providers reported seeing their PTSD patients did not vary by service branch ($p = 0.052$), but it did vary for MDD patients ($p < 0.05$). Specifically, Air Force providers saw their MDD patients more frequently than Navy providers ($p < 0.01$). All other comparisons between service branches were not statistically significant.

Summary

In this chapter, we focused on variables that could facilitate guideline-concordant care and variables that could be barriers to care. About three-quarters of MTF psychotherapy providers reported having received minimal training/supervision in at least one CPG-identified grade-A PTSD psychotherapy. The proportion was similar for MDD. Key informant discussions highlighted several service-level efforts to deliver training in evidence-based psychotherapies, so rates of endorsement could be a result of those efforts. It is notable, however, that our threshold of minimal training and supervision was set at a very low level, and many would argue that this threshold would not be sufficient to allow a provider to achieve competence in a given psychotherapy. Still, our survey results suggest that a quarter of MTF providers who deliver psychotherapy may not have the expertise to deliver *guideline-concordant* psychotherapy to their patients with PTSD. There were similar findings for MDD psychotherapy. Almost all psychiatrists/PNPs felt "very confident" in their ability to provide medication management to their patients with PTSD and MDD. However, with the exception of cognitive behavioral therapy for MDD, many psychotherapy providers expressed a lack of confidence in delivering evidence-based psychotherapies for PTSD and MDD. Fewer than half of psychotherapy providers felt "very confident" in their ability to deliver each of the grade-A psychotherapies for PTSD, and fewer than one-third felt very confident in their ability to deliver such treatments for uncomplicated MDD. The survey results suggest a need to continue increasing training, supervision, and consultation opportunities in guideline-concordant psychotherapies and to address barriers to obtaining training. Indeed, lack of protected time and travel support to attend professional trainings and workshops appeared to be the most prominent barriers, according to provider responses.

In terms of duration of treatment, most providers reported that they were able to see their PTSD and MDD patients for eight or more sessions; however, more than 15 percent indicated that they were unable to see their patients this often. Among psychotherapy-only providers, about half saw their PTSD and MDD patients weekly, with the remaining providers seeing patients less often. Among providers who delivered medication management only, nearly all providers saw their patients monthly or more often.

CHAPTER SIX

Summary and Recommendations

Overview

This report described the PH workforce at MTFs, examined the extent to which care for PTSD and MDD delivered in MTFs is consistent with VA/DoD CPGs, and identified facilitators and barriers to providing this care. Data sources included existing provider workforce data, a survey of more than 500 PH MTF providers, and semi-structured discussions with a small number of key informants. In this chapter, we highlight the strengths and limitations of our analyses, summarize our findings on the capacity of MTF providers to provide guideline-concordant care for patients with PTSD and MDD, and present policy recommendations and directions for future research.

Strengths and Limitations

This study had a number of key strengths. First, prior surveys of PH provider capacity have been limited to a single service branch (e.g., Wilk et al., 2013; Borah et al., 2013), but our survey included more than 500 PH providers across all service branches. Second, we included multiple provider types: psychiatrists, PNPs, doctoral-level psychologists, and master's-level clinicians. We were able to identify differences in practice and perceptions by service branch and provider type, thus increasing the utility of the survey findings for better targeting interventions to increase the use of guideline-concordant practices. Third, the fielded survey covered a wide range of domains, including how provider practices align with CPGs, training, and perceptions of barriers to care. This allowed us to develop a comprehensive picture of providers' perspectives on their capacity to deliver guideline-concordant PH care. Finally, we incorporated discussions with key informants from across DoD to provide context for our survey results.

The analyses presented in this report also have limitations, however. First, our overview of the provider workforce and the provider survey was limited to a selected group of PH provider types delivering care at MTFs. These specialty mental health providers included doctoral-level psychologists, master's-level clinicians, psychiatrists, and PNPs. Primary care providers (e.g., physicians, nurses) play an important role in treating PH conditions, but we did not examine the capacity of these providers to deliver guideline-concordant PH care. The population of patients with PTSD or MDD treated by specialty PH providers is likely different from the population treated by primary care providers; specifically, specialty PH providers may be more likely to treat a population whose PH conditions are more severe or who did not respond to initial treatment in primary care. Notably, however, 24 percent of PH providers who participated in our survey reported that they saw at least some of their PTSD and MDD patients in a primary care setting. We also did not include ancillary providers, such as chaplains, who may provide care for PH conditions outside the formal mental health system (Burnette, Ramchand, and Ayer, 2015). Relatedly, in our description of the PH provider workforce, our data did not address whether providers were full time or part time, the types of patients they treated (e.g., adults vs. children), or what proportion of their responsibilities were direct clinical service versus administrative. In addition, our analyses excluded contracted civilian personnel (who account for 18 percent of MTF PH providers and nearly 40 percent of Navy PH providers), and therefore, survey results cannot be generalized to the civilian contractor workforce. Further, we did not include purchased care providers that deliver care in the community that is paid for by the MHS through TRICARE. Our eligibility criterion of having seen a patient in the past 30 days is a strength in that it reduces recall bias; however, it also limits conclusions to actively practicing clinicians. Providers who only rarely see patients with MDD or PTSD (i.e., none in the past month) may provide care that differs from active MH providers.

Second, we drew our survey sample and contact information from the Defense Manpower Data Center's HMPDS. These data are updated annually, so they likely included some outdated or inaccurate provider and contact information. As a result, we may have missed some eligible providers or sampled some providers who should not have been included. Further, we did not know whether providers were actively seeing patients at the time of sampling and made this determination with a screening item at the time of survey completion. Each of these factors could have adversely affected our response rate. Still, our adjusted response rate is not unusual for provider surveys (39 percent), and we aimed to enhance our response rate by incorporating multiple forms of contact information. Specifically, email was our primary mode of contact, but we also attempted to reach providers via telephone and sent reminders via mail. Furthermore, we adjusted for nonresponse and weighted the sample to the target population of providers to improve the generalizability of our results.

Third, our survey data relied on provider self-reports; as a result, responses may have been incomplete or influenced by social desirability bias. In addition, two-thirds of providers reported that they did not access the selected patient's chart when responding to items about the most recent PTSD or MDD patient they had seen for psychotherapy or medication management. These providers' responses may be more subject to recall bias. While the items included in our survey assess important aspects of the providers' perspectives, these items have not been validated in terms of how they correspond with actual provider behavior. Furthermore, survey items assessed whether *currently* prescribed medications for PTSD and MDD were in accordance with VA/DoD CPGs, but we did not collect data on prior prescriptions for these PH conditions, psychopharmacological medications from other providers, or medications for medical conditions. Consequently, our findings capture only a snapshot of patient care. For example, if a provider reported a tricyclic antidepressant prescription for his or her most recent MDD patient, it is unclear whether it was prescribed as the first line of treatment or after the patient had tried other medications.

Fourth, to ensure adequate statistical power for provider-type comparisons, and due to their functionality as prescribers, we collapsed psychiatrists and PNPs into a single category. However, we are aware that these providers' education, training experiences, and responsibilities are quite different. Limited statistical power also prevented an examination of the interaction between service branch and provider type, which might have provided useful information.

Finally, we spoke with only 11 key informants. Due to the small number of informants and the brevity of these discussions (i.e., one hour), these discussions may not have fully captured the state of PH care, the organization of the PH workforce, or the scope of quality-improvement efforts across the MHS. Key informants may also have been unaware of or reluctant to disclose publicly specific challenges with implementation efforts experienced at individual MTFs.

Despite these limitations, this report provides a comprehensive picture of providers' perspectives on their capacity to deliver PH care within MTFs and presents detailed results by provider type and service branch. The remainder of this chapter highlights the primary findings from our study, followed by the policy implications of the findings.

Delivering Guideline-Concordant Care for PTSD and MDD in MTFs: Key Findings

Service Branches Rely on Different Mixes in Their PH Provider Workforce

The MHS is responsible for meeting the health and PH needs of 9.4 million beneficiaries; to do this, it employs close to 4,000 PH providers, including psychiatrists, PNPs, doctoral-level psychologists, master's-level psychologists, and clinical social workers who deliver care at MTFs. Across the service branches, master's-level clinicians make up the largest proportion (48 percent) of the PH workforce, including both master's-level psychologists and social workers. Doctoral-level psychologists make up 33 percent of the PH workforce, psychiatrists make up 15 percent, and PNPs make up 5 percent. Most PH providers are active-duty service members (37 percent) or civilian government employees (45 percent); contractors make up a small proportion of the workforce (18 percent).

Each service branch is responsible for managing its PH workforce and determining the appropriate mix of provider types across MTFs to best meet the needs of its beneficiary population (e.g., service members and dependents). As a result, there are some differences in workforce size and provider mix across service branches. At the population level, the Army has a ratio of PH providers to active-duty personnel more than twice as high as the other services, likely due to higher rates of some PH conditions among Army personnel. In terms of provider mix, the Air Force has a higher proportion of doctoral-level psychologists than the Army or Navy. There are also differences by service branch in how PH providers are employed; a higher proportion of Air Force providers are active-duty personnel (67 percent) compared with the Army (27 percent) or Navy (37 percent). The Navy is highly reliant on civilian contracted providers, who make up 38 percent of its PH workforce, compared with 6 and 24 percent of the Army and Air Force PH workforces, respectively.

Most Providers Reported Using Guideline-Concordant Psychotherapies, but Use Varied by Provider Type

Overall, 59 percent of psychotherapy providers identified a guideline-concordant psychotherapy as their primary approach for treatment for patients with PTSD. Psychologists (78 percent) were more likely than master's-level clinicians (56 percent), who, in turn, were more likely than psychiatrists/PNPs (21 percent) to indicate that they relied primarily on a guideline-concordant PTSD psychotherapy. Prescribers' use of supportive counseling as an adjunct to medication management (17 percent) may partially explain lower rates of delivery of CPG-endorsed psychotherapies among psychiatrists/PNPs, but it does not fully explain the gap between provider types. If we assume that all supportive counseling was an evidence-based adjunct to medication management among psychiatrists/PNPs, the rate (38 percent) would still trail that for psychologists (78 percent) and master's-level clinicians (56 percent). Across the services, Air Force providers were more likely than Army and Navy providers to select a CPG-concordant PTSD psychotherapy as their primary psychotherapy approach for PTSD. This may reflect the fact that all Air Force providers are required to be trained in evidence-based therapies for PTSD and undergo peer supervisions on a subset of their clinical cases. Although not all providers indicated that their primary PTSD psychotherapy approach was CPG-concordant, there nonetheless appeared to be a depth of familiarity with these approaches among master's-level clinicians and psychologists (e.g., 85 percent and 91 percent, respectively, reported ever having delivered a CPG-concordant psychotherapy).

Overall, 61 percent of psychotherapy providers identified a guideline-concordant psycho-therapy as their primary approach for treatment for patients with MDD. About two-thirds of psychologists (62 percent) and master's-level clinicians (67 percent) selected a guideline-concordant psychotherapy as their primary mode of treatment; fewer psychiatrists/PNPs did so (45 percent). However, a substantial majority of master's-level clinicians (90 percent), doctoral psychologists (94 percent), and psychiatrists/PNPs (79 percent) had delivered a guideline-concordant therapy for MDD in the past, which suggests that a lack of familiarity with these treatments may not be a primary barrier to delivering high-quality care for MDD.

Because a self-reported primary therapy approach may be most vulnerable to socially desirable responding, we asked about the specific techniques used with a patient as a means of indirectly assessing whether a guideline-concordant psychotherapy had been delivered. We hypothesized that this approach would be less influenced by social desirability. We expected that a smaller proportion of providers would report delivering all core elements of guideline-concordant psychotherapies than would indicate that a given psychotherapy was their primary approach. In fact, we found the opposite: Twice as many providers indicated that they had delivered all core cognitive processing therapy techniques than claimed that cognitive process-ing therapy was their primary psychotherapy approach, and three times as many providers indicated that they had delivered all core elements of eye movement desensitization and repro-cessing than claimed this therapy as their primary approach. It may be that the items designed to measure the core techniques of specific therapies instead captured relatively common therapy techniques shared across therapies. It should be noted, though, that relying upon items assess-ing use of psychotherapy techniques is early in its development as a means to measure quality.

Nearly All Psychiatrists and PNPs Reported Using Guideline-Concordant Medications to Treat PTSD and MDD, but Most Patients Received Multiple Psychopharmacologic Medications

Nearly 90 percent of psychiatrists/PNPs who had written prescriptions for their most recent PTSD patients prescribed at least one grade-A medication, and 97 prescribed at least one grade-A medication to their most recent MDD patient. Although reported use of grade-A medications was near the ceiling, there is some room for improvement: Among PTSD patients who were prescribed medication, 11 percent were receiving medications indicated as harmful to treatment progress in the VA/DoD *CPG for Post-Traumatic Stress* (grade D).

Finally, more research is needed to determine the appropriateness of prescribing practices for patients who receive multiple medications. Providers reported that 84 percent of PTSD patients were currently prescribed more than one medication, and nearly a quarter were currently prescribed four or more medications. Providers also indicated that 69 percent of MDD patients were currently prescribed more than one medication, with 12 percent receiving four or more. As the number of prescriptions goes up, the probability that any one of them is classified as a grade-A medication will also rise. This may partially explain the high reported rates of grade-A medication use.

Most Providers Reported Routinely Screening Patients for PTSD and MDD, but Fewer Used Validated Instruments to Monitor Treatment Outcomes

The majority of providers reported that either they or their support staff "always" screened for PTSD (71 percent) and MDD (79 percent) with a validated screening instrument. This may reflect the ongoing implementation of BHDP across MTFs, an outcome-monitoring system developed by the Army. We found differences across service branches in reported use of routine screening, but the results were not consistent. Army providers were significantly more likely than Air Force providers to screen new patients for PTSD with a validated screening instrument. However, this pattern was reversed for MDD, with Air Force providers more likely than both Army and Navy providers to report screening for MDD with a validated instrument.

These provider-reported screening rates are higher than findings from a medical record review of service members with PTSD or depression seen in the MHS (Hepner et al., 2017). Specifically, medical records for approximately 47 percent of service members beginning a new treatment episode for PTSD contained an assessment of symptom severity using the PTSD Checklist. Interestingly, 94 percent of these patients had an assessment for depression. Medical records for approximately 37 percent of service members beginning a new treatment episode for depression contained an assessment of symptom severity using the nine-item Patient Health Questionnaire. As BHDP implementation continues across MTFs, these screening rates will likely increase.

Comparatively fewer providers (58 percent) reported using a validated instrument of patient symptoms to inform treatment plan adjustments. Further, there was some variability by service branch, with Air Force providers more likely than Navy providers to use a validated patient symptom scale for this purpose.

The Majority of Therapists Reported Receiving at Least Minimal Training/Supervision in a Guideline-Concordant Psychotherapy, but Some Reported Difficulty Accessing Additional Training

The majority of providers who delivered psychotherapy (77 percent) reported that they had received minimally adequate training and supervision in at least one CPG-concordant psychotherapy for PTSD. The same was true for MDD psychotherapies (68 percent). We note that we established a lenient threshold for *minimally adequate training/supervision* to capture very low levels of this variable (at least eight hours of training and at least one hour of supervision). For training in PTSD psychotherapies, master's-level clinicians and psychologists were more likely to reach this threshold than were psychiatrists/PNPs. However, the pattern was different for MDD psychotherapy training, with psychologists and psychiatrist/PNPs more likely to reach the threshold than master's-level clinicians. There were no service differences in minimally adequate training in at least one CPG-concordant psychotherapy for either PTSD or MDD.

In general, psychotherapy providers were not highly confident in their ability to deliver grade-A PTSD psychotherapies. Fewer than half of providers (46 percent) felt very confident in their ability to deliver cognitive processing therapy, and this was the PTSD psychotherapy with the highest provider confidence level. A large cohort of providers (71 percent) felt very confident in their ability to deliver cognitive behavioral therapy for MDD, but providers were less confident in their ability to deliver interpersonal therapy and problem-solving therapy.

We found that confidence was significantly positively associated with receipt of minimally adequate training. This suggests that additional training could increase providers' confidence to deliver guideline-concordant PTSD and MDD psychotherapies; confidence may in turn increase delivery of these treatments. However, about one-quarter of providers reported that limits on travel and the lack of protected time affected their ability to access additional professional training.

Some Providers Reported Seeing Patients Infrequently

On average, MTF providers reported seeing 23 patients per week. For both psychologists and psychiatrists, these average weekly caseloads are consistent with averages reported among civilian providers. However, these visits may be stretched across more patients than for civilian providers. Indeed, one-quarter of providers strongly agreed with a statement indicating that they did not have the time in their schedule to see their patients as often as they would like. Almost half of therapists (specifically, providers who delivered psychotherapy but not medication) reported seeing their PTSD (45 percent) and MDD (49 percent) patients at least weekly, a typical scheduling frequency for psychotherapy patients. The remainder of these therapists saw their patients biweekly or less often. Most psychotherapies are tested using weekly sessions, and it remains unclear whether patients seen for psychotherapy visits less frequently than weekly receive the full benefit of the treatment. Ninety-five percent of prescribers (specifically, providers who prescribed medication but did not deliver psychotherapy) saw their patients at least monthly, a typical scheduling frequency for medication management patients.

It is important to consider whether providers are able to deliver an adequate course of treatment to patients. Most providers reported that they were able to see their PTSD patients (84 percent) and MDD patients (83 percent) for at least eight sessions. However, this means that 16–17 percent of providers typically saw their patients for fewer than eight sessions, a duration that may not be adequate to observe treatment response and recovery from MDD or PTSD. The duration over which prescribers saw their PTSD patients was not significantly different from that of therapists. However, therapists were more likely to indicate that they saw their MDD patients for 12 or more sessions. The survey data do not provide details about the reasons for short durations when present (e.g., scheduling difficulty, patient preference, symptom improvement). It is also important to note considerable variability in terms of recommended doses of psychotherapy. Although we set a lenient threshold of a minimum dose of eight sessions, note that the VA/DoD CPG provides specific sessions doses for different psychotherapies, some of which are significantly longer than eight sessions. For example, the recommended number of sessions for both cognitive behavioral therapy and interpersonal therapy is 16 to 20 (while the recommended length for problem-solving therapy is six sessions).

Recommendations to Guide Improvements in PH Care Across the MHS

Recommendation 1. Maximize the Effectiveness of Psychotherapy Training and Reduce Barriers

Recommendation 1a. Adopt a Systematic, Broad-Based Approach to Training and Certification in Guideline-Concordant Therapies, and Track Provider Progress

The majority of providers reported that their primary psychotherapy approach was a guideline-concordant therapy, and most providers met the threshold of receiving minimal training and supervision in at least one guideline-concordant therapy for PTSD and MDD. This may be a result of the multiple training efforts in evidence-based practices under way across service branches, as mentioned during multiple key informant discussions. As the MHS and service branches continue these efforts to increase implementation of guideline-concordant psychotherapy, it may be useful to adopt a systematic approach. While key informants described multiple training efforts, it appears there is no formal tracking system or provider certification process MHS-wide or by service branch to ensure that MTFs have the appropriate mix of provider competence to ensure availability of guideline-concordant psychotherapies. Certification in a particular type of psychotherapy indicates that a provider has received training and clinical supervision, and ultimately demonstrated competence in delivering that psychotherapy. This process is separate from the traditional credentialing process that ensures a provider has the appropriate degree and license. Academy of Cognitive Therapy provides a model for certification in cognitive behavioral therapy (Academy of Cognitive Therapy, 2016). Certification requirements should extend to all PH providers working in MTFs, including contracted providers.

Tracking provider certifications that indicate competence would allow service branches to target training efforts to particular providers or address a need for a particular type of psychotherapy. It should not be expected that a provider who delivers psychotherapy is competent in *all* grade-A psychotherapies for PTSD, yet it would be advantageous to know that an MTF has cognitive processing therapy, prolonged exposure, and eye movement and desensitization reprocessing psychotherapy available across their provider workforce. Patients may prefer a particular therapy or need to try an alternative after nonresponse to the therapy tried first. Tracking certification could also guide ongoing quality improvement. For example, this information could be used to populate a quality measure assessing the proportion of certified providers, with a goal of increasing the proportion of certified providers over time.

We found that some providers did not endorse a grade-A psychotherapy as their primary psychotherapy approach. Some had used a grade-A psychotherapy in the past, and some relied on psychotherapies that were not guideline concordant. Identifying and addressing provider-specific barriers to use of guideline-concordant therapies will be key strategies in improving quality of PH care.

Recommendation 1b. Reduce Barriers to Receiving Training in Guideline-Concordant Therapies

Among the multiple potential barriers to providing guideline-concordant treatment, assessed in the provider survey, barriers to training were the top two barriers. Specifically, providers reported that limits on travel and the lack of protected time affected their ability to access additional professional training. It is notable that our survey did not include contracted providers, and this is a group of providers typically not allowed to travel for trainings. Thus, the burden of travel restrictions for PH providers across the MHS may be even larger than suggested by our results. The MHS and service branch leadership should consider one or more of the following policy changes to increase access to trainings and reduce barriers to attending these trainings:

- Lift or reduce travel restrictions for training.
- Increase delivery of onsite trainings that do not require travel.
- Increase the use of web-based trainings.
- Provide protected time for attending trainings.

Over the course of the past several years, there has been a significant increase in the number of trainings for evidence-based therapies offered in virtual settings, thus limiting the need to travel to on-site sessions. At the same time, there may be accredited training offerings in the local MTF community (from non-DoD providers) that may also serve as alternatives. While these strategies would increase training opportunities, they may not address the second major training barrier identified, lack of protected time to participate in trainings. Providers may need additional support from their leadership to allow this protected time. This could be a challenge if provider incentives focus on number of patient visits rather than enhancing skills. Allowing for time to receive supervision/consultation following didactic training will help to ensure providers achieve competence in delivering the therapy, as research suggests that providers are not able to achieve competence with didactic workshops alone (Sholomskas et al., 2005).

Recommendation 2. Monitor the Frequency and Duration of Psychotherapy Treatment

Our results raised questions about whether PH providers are able to see patients with PTSD or MDD with the frequency and duration that may be associated with improved outcomes. When focused on therapists (specifically, providers who delivered psychotherapy, but not medication), less than half reported seeing their PTSD and MDD patients at least weekly, and the remainder saw their patients biweekly or less often. One-fifth reported that a typical course of treatment for patients with PTSD or MDD was fewer than eight sessions. This is notable when combined with our finding that a quarter of providers strongly agreed they did not have the time in their schedule to see their patients as often as they would like. While it is not clear that these results reflect lower-quality care, it highlights the importance of understanding these patterns to ensure access and availability to psychotherapy appointments. This finding, along with findings from a separate study in which MHS patients reported (Tanielian et al., 2016) frustration over not being able to get timely follow-up appointments, suggests that specific efforts to address the timeliness and frequency of psychotherapy visits are warranted.

Toward that end, the MHS should routinely monitor frequency and duration of psychotherapy treatment. This is consistent with recommendations from a recent RAND report (Hepner et al., 2016) that the MHS can improve at providing an adequate amount of treatment for service members beginning a new treatment episode for PTSD or depression. This report included data applying a quality measure that assessed whether service members received at least four psychotherapy visits or two medication management visits in the first eight weeks of beginning their treatment. A modified version of this measure could track frequency and duration of psychotherapy visits. Monitoring this measure would increase emphasis on timely ongoing appointments and balance existing incentives that focus on timely first appointments. While the optimum number and timing of visits are not certain, particularly for an individual patient, observing variation across providers, MTFs, and service branches and investigating the causes of these variations could guide quality improvement. Further, it would allow the MHS to gain a better understanding of the role that patient schedules, preferences, and response to treatment play in attenuating or increasing frequency and duration of treatment. Understanding "no shows" and cancellation rates may lead to implementation of proactive strategies to reduce these rates (e.g., reminder calls, no-show policies).

To the extent that the data reveal that capacity constraints are driving the inability to meet frequency and duration expectations, MHS leaders will need to consider options for expanding capacity and access (Tanielian et al., 2016). This could include additional expansion of telemental health opportunities, particularly using providers from other high quality locations, as well as by offering services during off-duty hours by either expanding clinic hours or utilizing centralized/off-site clinicians to deliver telemental health (Engel et al., 2016).

Recommendation 3. Expand Monitoring of Treatment Outcomes and Use That Information to Improve Quality of Care for PH Conditions

BHDP can support PH providers in using validated measures for both screening and monitoring clinical outcomes. Outcome monitoring across MTFs, using BHDP, is a promising effort that could be a core tool to monitor and improve outcomes. Providers reported using validated measures more frequently for screening than for informing adjustments to treatment. As the MHS works to increase monitoring of symptoms for patients with PH conditions, it will be important that providers understand how to use this information to inform treatment planning and adjustments to treatment. For example, providers may need additional training and feedback about how to use the information generated from BHDP at the patient level (e.g., patterns of symptoms over time that may suggest treatment needs to be adjusted or intensified). There is also the potential to augment BHDP with real time Clinical Decision Support tools and other technologies to help guide clinical decisionmaking and engage patients. Further, additional training and feedback could be used to ensure providers understand and evaluate their own practice. Encouraging providers to consider their own treatment outcomes, along with ways to improve (e.g., taking advantage of training opportunities), could engage providers in quality improvement.

In addition to engaging and training providers to effectively use BHDP in clinical practice, the MHS can expand use of BHDP data to guide quality improvement efforts. For example, these data could identify PH providers and MTFs that are "outliers" in terms of their ability to obtain improved outcomes (both higher performers and possible lower performers). Data that suggest some PH providers are lower performers should be interpreted with caution, as this method may identify experienced PH providers that MTFs rely on to treat their most challenging patients. These data could be linked with process quality measures that would indicate whether the care the provider delivers is typically guideline-concordant and consider whether care could be improved. For example, our analyses of primary psychotherapy approach suggested a small, but notable, proportion of providers endorsed types of psychotherapy that have not demonstrated effectiveness in treating PTSD or MDD (e.g., psychoanalysis, psychodynamic therapy). These PH providers could be tapped for training in guideline-concordant psychotherapies, which could lead to improved outcomes for them.

Recommendation 4. Develop a Systematic, MHS-Wide Approach to Increasing the Delivery of Guideline-Concordant PH Care Through a Continuous Quality Improvement Strategy

Because service branches have the responsibility for care delivery and staffing and training providers, there are few MHS-wide efforts to systematically monitor and improve PH care. BHDP is a notable exception and will provide visibility across the MHS on important aspects of the delivery of guideline-concordant care, including symptom monitoring and utilization. Key to increasing the capacity of the MHS to deliver such care, however, is developing and implementing system-wide continuous quality improvement efforts. While we are aware of several service branch–specific efforts, implementing MHS-wide efforts may increase efficiency and shared learning across the service branches. Although this report focused on care delivered by PH providers, these efforts should include care delivered to patients in primary care settings as well (i.e., including both primary care providers and PH providers integrated into primary care).

Monitoring the quality of care is a critical step in ensuring that all patients receive high-quality care. However, using the data effectively and systematically to implement quality improvement initiatives is equally important. By continuously gathering and using data at the system level, as recommended above, the MHS will be able to identify areas for improvement, develop and test strategies for improvement, and then implement those strategies across service branches. For example, this report identified variability in the extent to which PH providers have received training and supervision in guideline-concordant psychotherapies. While some service branches require all providers to receive training, the approach to training is not uniform. To address this, MHS leadership could develop an approach in conjunction with service branches and the Center for Deployment Psychology to ensure that all MHS providers who provide psychotherapy receive training and certification in one or more guideline-concordant psychotherapies. After implementing this approach, ongoing monitoring will provide necessary data to determine whether the approach was successful in increasing the proportion of providers certified in these psychotherapies, and, if not, to adjust the approach to better reach targeted providers.

To effectively implement systemic quality improvement efforts across the MHS, service branches and DHA will need to determine how to allocate responsibility for these efforts and to assure that those accountable for quality at each level (from MTF to service branch) receive appropriate training in quality improvement tools and procedures. While DHA is collecting data and monitoring quality across service branches, past efforts to improve care have occurred within service branches, rather than across the MHS as a whole. We recommend that MHS policymakers consider mechanisms for system-wide improvements, which should increase efficiency and reduce variability in the delivery of care.

Directions for Future Research

The analyses presented in this report provide results that can guide the MHS in targeting efforts to improve quality of care for PTSD and depression. These analyses also raised some questions, so here we outline several high-priority research directions.

- Describe perceptions and practices of contract PH providers. We were not able to include them in our provider survey, but they make up a significant portion of the provider workforce (18 percent). Contractors are an even larger proportion of the Navy's workforce (38 percent).

- Describe perceptions and practices of purchased care providers. We were not able to include community providers contracted to provide care paid for by the MHS through TRICARE. These providers are an important part of the MHS, yet the MHS has little awareness of the quality of care delivered by these providers or the barriers and facilitators to delivering guideline-concordant care.

- Assess perceptions and practices of primary care providers to understand how they manage PH conditions and identify any specific training requirements or other quality improvement needs. Given the reliance upon primary care settings to address PH conditions, particularly within some service branches, this work will be critical to ensuring that no matter the setting, MHS patients will be afforded the opportunity to receive high-quality care for PTSD and MDD (Batka et al., 2016).

- Describe the distribution and composition of the PH provider workforce at the MTF level to better understand the settings (e.g., inpatient, ambulatory) in which these providers work. As PH providers can work in multiple settings, understanding the number and type of providers working in each setting can help inform assessments of capacity and better target interventions aimed at improving the quality of care.

- Understand prescribing patterns to identify potential problematic polypharmacy, including benzodiazepine use. Similar to prior work, data suggest that patients with PTSD or depression receive multiple psychopharmacologic medications (also, potentially, other medications for non-PH conditions) and the appropriateness of this complex prescribing is unclear.

- Assess service member and provider attitudes and use of BHDP to inform approaches to increase meaningful clinical use of outcome data.

This study expanded on previous RAND work on quality of care for PH conditions by describing the PH workforce at MTFs, examining the extent to which MTF providers report care for PTSD and MDD that is consistent with clinical practice guidelines, and identifying facilitators and barriers to providing this care. These findings highlight areas of strength for the MHS, as well as areas that should be targeted for quality improvement. The results presented here can inform how the MHS and service branches can support continuous improvement in the PH care the MHS delivers.

Survey Sampling and Weighting

Chapter Two provides an overview of the approach used for sampling and weighting. In this appendix, we provide additional details regarding our approach.

Survey Sampling

In this section, we provide an overview of survey sampling in Chapter Two. Table A.1 shows the breakdown of the population of providers. The table also stratifies the population on the basis of provider employment status (active-duty service member or civilian), in addition to service and level of education. We did not distinguish providers on the basis of their employment status in our analyses because we were not powered to include an additional stratum; however, we made this distinction during sampling (e.g., active-duty and civilian providers were sampled at different rates in certain cases).

Unfortunately, we were unable to obtain valid contact information for all providers in the population outlined in Table A.1. Specifically, we could not obtain email addresses for several providers, and this was a necessary mode of contact for our operations. The prevalence of missing email addresses was small, however. In total, 89.6 percent of the population had an email address, and this rate did not vary noticeably across the strata. The sampled providers (i.e., those selected to be contacted for participation in our study) were drawn from only those who had email addresses. Nonetheless, our sampling strategy and weighting approaches are illustrated in a manner that presumes that all providers in the population were eligible to be sampled (and that any unavailability of email addresses occurred randomly and not systematically). This ensured that our final cohort of respondents, when weighted, would be representative of all providers and not just those with email addresses.

Sampling Strategy

Under the objectives and restrictions described previously, we sampled from the population outlined in Table A.1 at rates shown in Table A.2. Note that the percentages in Table A.2 are given as a portion of the full provider population (those who did and did not have email addresses). In several strata, we sampled all available providers.

Response and Eligibility Rates

When a provider accessed the survey, he or she was asked to complete a single screening item to determine eligibility for the survey. We do not know which nonrespondents (those who did not complete the screener) were eligible to participate. Therefore, we cannot determine the rate at which sampled providers responded to our survey out of only those who were eligible.

Table A.1
Number of Providers in the Provider Population, by Stratum

Active-Duty Service Member	Army	Navy	Air Force	Total
Psychiatrist	135	110	80	325
Psychiatric nurse practitioner	41	38	31	110
Psychologist (doctoral-level)	194	99	205	498
Psychologist (master's-level)	0	0	0	0
Social worker	270	85	243	598
Total	640	332	559	1,531

Civilian	Army	Navy	Air Force	Total
Psychiatrist	137	34	4	175
Psychiatric nurse practitioner	39	11	0	50
Psychologist (doctoral-level)	396	87	23	506
Psychologist (master's-level)	93	9	1	103
Social worker	914	84	40	1,038
Total	1,579	225	68	1,872

Total (Active-Duty and Civilian Providers)	Army	Navy	Air Force	Total
Psychiatrist	272	144	84	500
Psychiatric nurse practitioner	80	49	31	160
Psychologist (doctoral-level)	590	186	228	1,004
Psychologist (master's-level)	93	9	1	103
Social worker	1,184	169	283	1,636
Total	2,219	557	627	3,403

However, to help illustrate the propensity for sampled providers to agree to participate in our study, Table A.3 shows the percentage of providers who completed the screener within each stratum. The overall rate of screener completion was 45.5 percent. We observed comparatively poor rates of screener completion (around 40 percent) among master's-level psychologists and social workers, as well providers from the Army, and we observed comparatively high rates (around 50 percent) among doctoral-level psychologists and providers from the Navy. These values may underestimate the true rate of response among eligible providers, as providers may have been able to determine that they were ineligible prior to completing the screener and may consequentially have chosen not to participate.

The responding providers who screened as being eligible for the survey were given the full survey; our final analytic cohort consisted of eligible providers who completed the survey. The breakdown of the analytic cohort by sample stratum is shown in Table A.4. Completion rates were high overall, with only six providers screened as being eligible being excluded from the

Table A.2
Proportion of Providers Sampled from Each Stratum

Active-Duty Service Member	Army	Navy	Air Force	Total
Psychiatrist (%)	62.2	98.2	87.5	80.6
Psychiatric nurse practitioner (%)	92.7	94.7	83.9	90.9
Psychologist (doctoral-level) (%)	18.0	66.7	55.1	43.0
Psychologist (master's-level) (%)	—	—	—	—
Social worker (%)	14.1	61.2	67.9	42.6
Total (%)	30.5	78.9	66.9	54.3

Civilian	Army	Navy	Air Force	Total
Psychiatrist (%)	72.3	79.4	75.0	73.7
Psychiatric nurse practitioner (%)	89.7	90.9	—	90.0
Psychologist (doctoral-level) (%)	20.5	47.1	56.5	26.7
Psychologist (master's-level) (%)	66.7	66.7	100.0	67.0
Social worker (%)	20.2	77.4	75.0	27.0
Total (%)	29.3	66.2	69.1	35.1

Total (Active-Duty and Civilian Providers)	Army	Navy	Air Force	Total
Psychiatrist (%)	67.3	93.8	86.9	78.2
Psychiatric nurse practitioner (%)	91.3	93.9	83.9	90.6
Psychologist (doctoral-level) (%)	19.7	57.5	55.3	34.8
Psychologist (master's-level) (%)	66.7	66.7	100.0	67.0
Social worker (%)	18.8	69.2	68.9	32.7
Total (%)	29.6	73.8	67.1	43.8

final cohort. Rates of eligibility were high as well (77 percent of participants who responded to the screener were eligible), but this rate did not vary markedly by stratum. There was some variation in eligibility rates by provider type (82 percent of prescribing providers were eligible and 72 percent of master's-level psychologists and social workers were eligible); there was no discernable difference in eligibility rates by service branch.

Our final cohort consisted of 520 of the 1,489 sampled providers, giving us a raw response rate of 35.9 percent. The 969 nonrespondents included providers who were ineligible and those for whom we had invalid contact information, in addition to those who refused to participate.

Weighting

Data were weighted to ensure that the final analytic sample was representative of the full population of providers relevant to this study. To account for the potential lack of representativeness,

Table A.3
Proportion of Sampled Providers Who Responded to the Eligibility Screening Item

Active-Duty Service Member	Army	Navy	Air Force	Total
Psychiatrist (%)	41.7	52.8	47.1	47.7
Psychiatric nurse practitioner (%)	39.5	50.0	50.0	46.0
Psychologist (doctoral-level) (%)	51.4	53.0	52.2	52.3
Psychologist (master's-level) (%)	—	—	—	—
Social worker (%)	47.4	44.2	47.9	47.1
Total (%)	44.1	50.8	49.2	48.5

Civilian	Army	Navy	Air Force	Total
Psychiatrist (%)	40.4	59.3	33.3	44.2
Psychiatric nurse practitioner (%)	45.7	60.0	—	48.9
Psychologist (doctoral-level) (%)	48.1	63.4	38.5	51.9
Psychologist (master's-level) (%)	32.3	50.0	0.0	33.3
Social worker (%)	34.1	50.8	20.0	36.4
Total (%)	38.5	56.4	25.5	41.6

Total (Active-Duty and Civilian Providers)	Army	Navy	Air Force	Total
Psychiatrist (%)	41.0	54.1	46.6	46.5
Psychiatric nurse practitioner (%)	42.5	52.2	50.0	46.9
Psychologist (doctoral-level) (%)	49.1	57.0	50.8	52.1
Psychologist (master's-level) (%)	32.3	50.0	0.0	33.3
Social worker (%)	36.3	47.9	43.6	41.5
Total (%)	40.2	52.8	46.6	45.5

NOTE: Includes providers who were deemed ineligible; N = 1,489.

we weighted the data in two ways. First, we needed to account for the sampling design because we oversampled from various strata of providers. Second, we needed to account for survey nonresponse. Sampled providers who responded may have been systematically different from those who did not, leading to an analytic sample that would not represent the population. Therefore, to account for each of these potential sources of bias, we calculated two sets of weights: design weights and nonresponse weights. The final weights were the product of each of these sets.

Design Weights

Design weights account for differential rates of sampling that are a consequence of the sample design. To calculate design weights, one determines each sampled provider's probability of being sampled. For sampling, the provider population was divided into 15 strata on the basis of service branch (Army, Navy, and Air Force) and provider type (psychiatrist, psychiatric

Table A.4
Analytic Cohort, by Stratum

Active-Duty Service Members	Army	Navy	Air Force	Total
Psychiatrist	29	47	27	103
Psychiatric nurse practitioner	12	15	12	39
Psychologist (doctoral-level)	15	25	44	84
Psychologist (master's-level)	0	0	0	0
Social worker	14	16	61	91
Total	70	103	144	317

Civilians	Army	Navy	Air Force	Total
Psychiatrist	32	16	1	49
Psychiatric nurse practitioner	12	2	0	14
Psychologist (doctoral-level)	32	20	3	55
Psychologist (master's-level)	12	0	0	12
Social worker	45	24	4	73
Total	133	62	8	203

Total (Active-Duty and Civilian Providers)	Army	Navy	Air Force	Total
Psychiatrist	61	63	28	152
Psychiatric nurse practitioner	24	17	12	53
Psychologist (doctoral-level)	47	45	47	139
Psychologist (master's-level)	12	0	0	12
Social worker	59	40	65	164
Total	203	165	152	520

NOTE: N = 520.

nurse practitioners, doctoral-level psychologists, master's-level psychologists, and social workers). Since providers were sampled randomly within each stratum, the sampling probability for each provider in a specific stratum was equal to the number of providers sampled from that stratum divided by the total number of providers in that stratum. Ultimately, we sampled only providers who had valid email addresses. When we use the total number of providers in a stratum in the calculation of sampling probabilities, we are effectively assuming that email addresses were missing at random within strata. Diagnostics performed on the population support this conclusion. Table A.2 shows the sampling probabilities for providers in each stratum. A provider's design weight is equal to the inverse of his or her selection probability.

Nonresponse Weights

Nonresponse weights were assigned to each respondent. Sampled providers interested in participating in the survey were first screened to determine whether they were eligible. Of the 677 providers who expressed interest, 151 were ineligible because they indicated that they had not provided psychiatric treatment to an adult patient with PTSD or MDD at an MTF in the previous 30 days. Another six providers were excluded for other reasons. We do know which nonresponding providers were ineligible. Therefore, we treated all providers who completed the screening item as respondents (regardless of whether or not they were determined to be eligible). Calculating nonresponse rates involves approximating each sampled provider's probability of being a respondent versus a nonrespondent.

There was also a possibility that the likelihood of response was dependent on characteristics not included in our sampling frame. Therefore, we calculated a logistic regression model that used an indicator of a provider's status as a respondent or nonrespondent as the outcome variable and provider characteristics as predictor variables. Characteristics must have been observed for all sampled providers (not just respondents) to be included in this nonresponse model. Variables in the nonresponse model included provider type, service branch, employment status (active-duty service member or government civilian), gender, and geographical census division (e.g., New England, Mid-Atlantic, South Atlantic). Since we used strata based on an interacted version of provider type, service branch, and employment status for sampling (see Table A.2), we also used interactions of these variables in our nonresponse model.

Model selection was used to include only predictors that informed the nonresponse weights (as well as interactions). The final model included service branch, gender, and an interaction of an overseas indicator (based on geographical division) and military status. A provider's response probability was set as the predicted value from this logistic regression. The nonresponse weight for each responding provider is the inverse of his or her response probability.

Final Weights

Final weights for each provider classified as a respondent were the product of the provider's design weight and nonresponse weight. Providers who screened as being ineligible and other responding providers later determined to not be eligible for the study were dropped from all analyses (despite the fact that they were assigned a final weight)—no weights were modified as a result of these exclusions. In doing this, we effectively assumed that, within each stratum, a provider's likelihood of responding did not depend on his or her status as being eligible or ineligible. Upon excluding ineligible providers, our pool of respondents, when weighted using the final weights, was representative of the population of providers eligible for our study.

Using the final weights, we found the approximate design effect for the full sample to be 1.68, which implies that the effective sample size for the full sample was 310. Therefore, estimators found using the complete weighted sample have a maximum margin of error of 5.6 percent. The moderate design effect is a consequence of oversampling from certain strata; the design effect within strata is lower (e.g., for Navy providers only, the design effect is 1.10, and the effective sample size of Navy providers is 150, which yields a maximum margin of error of 8 percent). Even when weighted, these samples are sufficient for comparison on the basis of provider type or service branch. Specifically, comparisons of Army to Navy providers have a minimum detectable effect size with 80-percent power (in terms of Cohen's d) of 0.324 (which is a small to medium effect size).

Survey Domains

This appendix provides a description of the survey domains used in this study and details which respondents viewed and responded to particular items. Where appropriate, the appendix also includes information on the variables created from these survey domains for data analysis.

Provider Characteristics

Respondents provided information about their race and ethnicity (Office of Management and Budget, 2006), along with their years in practice. The survey was programmed to deliver these items to all respondents who had delivered PTSD/MDD services in the past 30 days.

Professional characteristics were collected on the survey and were available through the HMPDS data, including provider type (e.g., clinical psychologist, PNP), military status (e.g., active component, DoD government civilian), and service branch. Provider self-report and HMPDS data were largely concordant, so we present only the HMPDS data for these variables.

Theoretical Orientation

To assess providers' primary and secondary theoretical orientations, we included a survey item from the American Psychological Association Division 29's survey of psychotherapists, which lists 12 options and includes a free-response field (Norcross and Rogan, 2013). Respondents selected their primary and secondary orientations from a list that included, for example, behavioral, interpersonal, and psychoanalytic. Because our sample included psychiatrists and PNPs, who may not identify with a psychotherapy theoretical orientation, we added "biological" as a response option. Respondents who indicated they had delivered care to an adult patient with MDD or PTSD in the past 30 days (i.e., active PTSD or MDD providers) viewed and responded to this item.

Practice Characteristics

We developed eight items to assess providers' practice characteristics. Respondents provided information on their average number of patient visits per week (for all patients) and the number of these visits conducted in a primary care setting. In addition, providers reported the percentage of their patients with PTSD and the percentage of patients with MDD in their current patient caseload. Finally, providers reported their average number of visits with PTSD/MDD patients during a typical course of treatment and the frequency of these visits. The survey was programmed to deliver these items to active PTSD or MDD providers.

Measurement-Based Care

Measurement-based care is an approach in which clinical data are used to inform patient treatment (Harding et al., 2011). Routine, standardized assessment of symptoms not only allows clinicians to monitor patient response to treatment (and modify care as necessary), but also gives administrators insight into patient treatment outcomes on a systemic level. Three items captured the use of measurement-based care in providers' practice settings and were programmed so that all active PTSD and MDD providers viewed and responded to them. Participants detailed how often structured instruments were used to screen for PTSD or depression and to inform changes to patient treatment plans. Providers responded on a five-point scale that ranged from "never" to "always."

Psychotherapy Approaches for PTSD and MDD

We assessed the types of psychotherapy approaches (sometimes referred to as *treatment modalities*) that providers used with patients with PTSD or MDD. Screening questions were used to ensure that only providers who deliver psychotherapy for PTSD viewed and responded to questions about PTSD psychotherapy, and only providers who deliver psychotherapy for MDD viewed and responded to questions about MDD psychotherapy. The program skipped all other providers past these modules.

Providers who had a therapy session with at least one patient with PTSD in the previous 30 days were asked to indicate the therapy types they used to treat patients with the condition. Participants reported on all treatment modalities ever provided to a PTSD patient and then specified their "primary mode of therapy" for patients with PTSD. The checklist of 29 therapies included guideline-concordant therapies for PTSD (e.g., cognitive processing therapy), guideline-concordant therapies for other conditions (e.g., interpersonal therapy), and ineffective or untested therapies (e.g., existential). We also created dichotomous variables to assess whether the provider had delivered any of the psychotherapies strongly recommended for PTSD in the CPG for Post-Traumatic Stress (i.e., cognitive processing therapy, prolonged exposure, eye movement reprocessing and desensitization, and stress inoculation training) and whether they chose one of the strongly recommended psychotherapies as their primary psychotherapy approach for patients with PTSD.

Respondents who indicated they had provided therapy to a patient with MDD in the previous 30 days completed a series of questions similar to those described for PTSD patients. Respondents selected all treatment modalities ever provided to an MDD patient and specified their primary approach. We created dichotomous variables to assess whether the provider had delivered any of the psychotherapies strongly recommended in the CPG for MDD as a first-line psychotherapy for uncomplicated MDD (i.e., cognitive behavioral therapy, interpersonal therapy, and problem-solving therapy) and whether they chose one of the strongly recommended psychotherapies as their primary approach for patients with MDD.

Psychotherapy Techniques for PTSD and MDD

The psychotherapy technique modules instructed providers who had delivered PTSD psychotherapy in the past 30 days to use their electronic charting system (if available) to identify their most recent adult patient with PTSD. Once the patient was identified, providers selected any comorbid psychiatric diagnoses within broad classes (e.g., substance use disorder) and indicated the number of visits completed.

Using this patient as a reference, the subset of survey respondents completed an 18-item session behavior scale (adapted from Wilk et al., 2013) that assessed provider use of therapeutic techniques associated with the three VA/DoD CPG-endorsed therapies for PTSD: (1) prolonged exposure, (2) cognitive processing therapy, and (3) eye movement desensitization and reprocessing. Six items assessed core techniques of prolonged exposure (e.g., "How often did you ask this patient to recount the traumatic event(s) aloud repeatedly, including telling you the details of the event, their thoughts and feelings?"). Five items assessed core techniques of cognitive processing therapy (e.g., "How often did you assign self-monitoring homework to identify the connection between events, thoughts, and feelings?"). Four items assessed core techniques of eye movement desensitization and reprocessing (e.g., "How often did you ask this patient to focus on the traumatic image, negative thoughts, and body sensations while moving his/her eyes back and forth to laterally track your finger?"). We adapted the scale by adding two "distractor" items that assessed psychodynamic techniques (e.g., "How often did you explore the deeper emotional meaning of this patient's concerns of behaviors?") (Hepner et al., 2010). We also changed the original response options (yes/no) to a six-point scale that ranged from 1 (never used the technique) to 6 (always used the technique) during sessions with the most recent PTSD patient. Any response other than "never" was coded as having delivered the treatment technique, and we calculated the percentage of providers who had delivered all core therapeutic techniques for each approach. Psychometric properties were not reported for this measure.

We measured MDD psychotherapy providers' adherence to CPG recommendations for MDD using a modified version of the Psychotherapy Practice Scale: Clinician Depression Care (Hepner et al., 2010). Our revised version of the instrument included three subscales that assessed providers' use of techniques unique to cognitive behavioral therapy (five items; for example, "How often did you help this patient understand the beliefs and assumptions behind their thinking [e.g., core beliefs, cognitive schemas]?"), interpersonal therapy (four items; for example, "How often did you examine the emotional response the patient had during interpersonal interactions?"), and psychodynamic therapy (two items). While endorsement of cognitive behavioral therapy and interpersonal therapy techniques signify fidelity to MDD CPG recommendations, use of psychodynamic therapy methods indicates deviance from these guidelines (Management of Major Depressive Disorder Working Group, 2009). Responses were recorded on a six-point scale ranging from 1 (never used the technique) to 6 (always used the technique) during sessions with the most recent MDD patient. The scale did not include session behaviors associated with stress inoculation training, an effective but uncommon therapy for MDD. Psychometric properties for the original scale were good, with subscale internal reliability ranging from $\alpha = 0.79$ to $\alpha = 0.84$ and subscales supported with confirmatory factor analysis (Hepner et al., 2010). Scale scores were computed by averaging responses across all items assessing a given technique and then converting the means to a t-score. A t-score is a standardized score with a mean of 50 and standard deviation of 10.

Medication Management for PTSD and MDD

The medication management modules were programmed for delivery only to providers who delivered a medication management visit in the past 30 days.

Providers who had seen a PTSD patient for a medication management in the past 30 days were presented with a survey prompt to use their electronic charting system (if available) to identify their most recent adult patient with PTSD. Once the patient was identified, this group of prescribers indicated any comorbid psychiatric diagnoses within broad classes (e.g., substance use disorder). If the patient was receiving any psychopharmacologic medications as of his or her last visit, respondents provided the name and dosage of scheduled, depot (by injection, typically long acting), and PRN (as-needed) psychopharmacologic medications currently prescribed to the patient.

In the second medication management section, providers who had seen a patient with MDD in the previous 30 days went through a parallel process of identifying the most recent patient, describing comorbid conditions, and listing all currently prescribed psychopharmacologic medications. These items were adapted from the Army Behavioral Health Practice and Treatment Study (Wilk et al., 2013).

For this report, all medication names were coded into classes of medication (e.g., hypnotics, antidepressants). Medication names were also coded into the grades specified in the VA/DoD *CPG for Post-Traumatic Stress* (Management of Post-Traumatic Stress Working Group, 2010). Grade-A medications for PTSD included SSRIs and SNRIs (strong recommendation). Grade-B medications included mirtazapine, prazosin, tricyclic antidepressants, nefazodone, and monoamine oxidase inhibitors (MAOIs) (i.e., "at least fair evidence of effectiveness"). Grade-D medications included tiagabine, guanfacine, valproate, topiramate, and risperidone ("at least fair evidence that the intervention is ineffective"). Finally, benzodiazepines are also included as grade-D medication for PTSD, but they are additionally described as harmful in that they could worsen PTSD outcomes. We created a separate grade-D class to describe ineffective drugs that are also potentially harmful.

For MDD, we coded medications into grade-A medications recommended for first-line treatment of uncomplicated MDD: SSRIs, SNRIs, bupropion, and mirtazapine (Management of Major Depressive Disorder Working Group, 2009). Grade-B medications for MDD included nortriptyline and tricyclic antidepressants.

Training, Supervision, and Confidence in Guideline-Concordant Treatments for PTSD and MDD

To measure system capacity to deliver evidence-based treatment for PTSD and MDD, we assessed the degree to which MHS providers (who had delivered PTSD or MDD care in the past 30 days) had received training and supervision in evidence-based approaches and whether they felt confident in delivering these treatments. Although some providers with adequate training to deliver evidence-based care may choose to instead deliver an untested or ineffective therapy, their training nonetheless represents untapped capacity in the system to deliver effective care.

We assessed formal training in evidence-based treatment for PTSD and MDD with an item adapted from the Army Behavioral Health Practice and Treatment Study (Wilk et al., 2013). Providers indicated the number of hours (none, one to eight hours, more than eight hours) of formal training they had received in the five treatments for PTSD recommended in the VA/DoD *CPG for Post-Traumatic Stress* (i.e., medication management, prolonged exposure, cognitive processing therapy, eye movement desensitization and reprocessing, and stress inoculation training) (Management of Post-Traumatic Stress Working Group, 2010) and the four treatments for MDD recommended in the VA/DoD CPG for that condition (i.e., medication management, interpersonal therapy, cognitive behavioral therapy, and problem-solving therapy) (Management of Major Depressive Disorder Working Group, 2009). Formal training as defined included classes, workshops, lecture series, seminars, and webinars.

Given evidence suggesting that direct supervision is a necessary ingredient to ensure that providers offer evidence-based treatments with fidelity to the tested model (Sholomskas et al., 2005), we included an item to assess the number of hours of direct supervision or consultation (none, one to eight hours, nine to 20 hours, more than 20 hours) that providers reported receiving in each of the VA/DoD-recommended treatments for PTSD and MDD (Management of Major Depressive Disorder Working Group, 2016; Management of Post-Traumatic Stress Working Group, 2010). Supervision or consultation was defined as supervision received from an expert clinician beyond a workshop or class. From these items, we constructed dichotomous "minimally adequate training/supervision" variables for each treatment type, defined as having received more than eight hours of training and at least one hour of supervision in a given modality. Finally, providers rated their confidence level in delivering each evidence-based treatment on a four-point scale (not at all confident, somewhat confident, moderately confident, or very confident). In this report, we describe the percentage of providers who indicated that they were "very confident" delivering a given treatment modality.

Barriers to Implementing Guideline-Concordant Care

We evaluated barriers to delivering care for PTSD and MDD at both the provider and facility levels. We included 26 items, adapted from multiple questionnaires, to assess barriers across 11 domains (Aarons et al., 2012; American Psychiatric Association, 1996; Borah et al., 2013; Center for Deployment Psychology, 2013; Maslach, Jackson and Leiter, 1996; Meredith et al., 1999). To avoid response bias, we worded some barrier items in the opposite direction, such that they indicated facilitators. We examined respondents' attitudes toward research, provider attitudes toward standardized practices, provider autonomy to deliver any treatment versus provider accountability for delivering CPG-concordant care, provider caseload, provider burnout, beliefs that all psychotherapies are equally effective, impact of military systems on patient ability to receive appropriate care, provider ability to acquire additional training, provider openness to learning new treatments, perceptions of patient-centered care (versus standardized CPG-concordant care), availability of training and supervision resources, providers' degree of communication with patients' commanders, and facility support for measurement-based care. These items were rated on a scale that ranged from 1 (strongly disagree) to 5 (strongly agree). For items phrased as barriers, "strongly agree" indicated that it was perceived to be a substantial barrier for the provider. In contrast, for items phrased as facilitators, "strongly disagree" indicated that it was a substantial barrier for the provider. We dichotomized these responses to highlight substantial barriers relative to other response options.

Survey of Psychological Heath Providers in the MHS

Phone Introductory Script

Hello, this is _____ calling on behalf of RAND Corporation. May I please speak to **John Doe?**

[IF ASKED WHAT YOU ARE CALLING ABOUT BY GATEKEEPER] We are following up on an email invitation to participate in a survey about clinical care for service members with PTSD or MDD. We're hoping to learn more about the resources available to military providers and the challenges they face. This request was approved by the Army Human Research Protections Office.

[ONCE PROPER RESPONDENT ON PHONE SAY] Hello, my name is _____. I am calling from Davis Research regarding a survey that the RAND Corporation is conducting. You may have recently received an email invitation to participate in a survey about clinical care for service members with PTSD or MDD. We're hoping to learn more about the resources available to military providers and the challenges they face.

If you agree to participate, the survey will take approximately 30 minutes to complete. If you are off-duty, when you complete the survey, we will provide a **$50** gift card to Amazon, Starbucks or PayPal as a token of appreciation for your time.

Caring for PTSD and Depression Within the Military Health System

You have been invited to participate in a survey about clinical care for service members with PTSD or depression. We also hope to learn more about the resources available to military providers and the challenges they face.

The RAND Corporation, a private, non-profit research institution, is conducting this project, which is funded by the Defense Centers of Excellence for Psychological Health and Traumatic Brain Injury (DCoE).

The survey will take approximately 20 minutes to complete online, or 30 minutes by telephone. While there is no direct benefit for participating in this project, our findings could lead to improvements in the psychological health care that individuals receive at MHS facilities in the future. If you complete the survey during off-duty time, we will provide a $50 Amazon gift card, a $50 Starbucks gift card, or a $50 PayPal credit as a token of appreciation. Providers may also complete the survey during duty time, if they decline the gift card incentive.

Your participation in this survey is entirely voluntary. If you do decide to participate, you can skip questions or stop taking the survey at any time.

Risks of participation are minimal. You will not be asked to provide sensitive information, and we will protect the confidentiality of your responses. Only project personnel will have access to the information you provide. RAND will not include participant names in any reports. The RAND Corporation's Human Subjects Protection Committee and the Army Human Research Protection Office have reviewed and approved the study procedures. Representatives of the DoD are authorized to review our research records.

The DoD Privacy Advisory states that the Defense Manpower Data Center has provided certain information about you to allow RAND to conduct this survey. Your name and contact information have been used to send you notifications and information about this survey. The Defense Manpower Data Center has provided certain demographic information to reduce the number of questions in the survey and minimize the burden on your time. Your response and demographic data are linked by RAND to allow for a thorough analysis of the responses by demographics. RAND has not been authorized by DoD to identify or link survey response and demographic information with your name and contact information. The resulting reports will not include analysis of groupings of less than 15.

We would be happy to answer any questions you might have about the study or your participation. For more information about this survey, you may contact:
Kimberly Hepner, Ph.D.
Senior Behavioral Scientist, RAND Corporation
Tel: (310) 393-0411 ext. 6381
Email: hepner@rand.org

If you have any questions or concerns about your rights as a research participant, you may also contact the Human Subjects Protection Committee at RAND, 1776

Main Street, P.O. Box 2138, Santa Monica, CA 90407-2138, (310) 393-0411, ext. 6369.

Please indicate whether you consent to participate in this study:
☐ Yes, I agree to participate
☐ I do not want to participate in this study and I would like to exit the survey now.

Eligibility Screen

<Following informed consent language> Before beginning, we need to see if this study applies to you and your work.

WEB

S1. <u>In the last 30 days</u>, have you provided *psychiatric treatment* to an adult patient with Major Depressive Disorder (or MDD) *or* PTSD at a Military Treatment Facility? Psychiatric treatment includes counseling, psychotherapy, or medication management for MDD or PTSD. A Military Treatment Facility includes any military hospital or clinic including primary or specialty care clinics and "aid station" style settings.

TELEPHONE

In the last 30 days, have you provided psychiatric treatment to an adult patient with Major Depressive Disorder (or MDD) or PTSD at a Military Treatment Facility?

Psychiatric treatment includes counseling, psychotherapy, or medication management for MDD or PTSD. A Military Treatment Facility includes any military hospital or clinic including primary or specialty care clinics and "aid station" style settings.

○ No
○ Yes

[Require respondents to answer this question. Do NOT allow skip.]

[Programming Note: If S1 = 'No", then skip to Ineligible screen.]

Ineligible Screen Text: Based on your response, it appears that you did not treat an adult patient with one of these conditions in the last month (at a military treatment facility). The survey that follows focuses on treatment of patients with one of these conditions. Therefore, there are no further questions for you to answer.

We thank you for you service to the military and your willingness to participate in this survey. At this time, you are not eligible to participate.

Thank you.

> You are eligible to participate in this survey. As you answer these questions, please consider only treatment that you delivered at a military treatment facility. Please <u>exclude</u> the care you deliver in other settings, such as a private practice or non-military clinic or hospital.
>
> It is not necessary to have access to your patient notes or AHLTA to complete the survey. However, if available, access to AHLTA will simplify your response to some questions.
>
> **WEB**
>
> We will not request any personally identifying or HIPPA protected information about your patients.
>
> **TELEPHONE**
>
> I will not request any personally identifying or HIPAA protected information about your patients.

Practice Characteristics

For all remaining items, allow respondents to skip past them without answering the question. Unless otherwise specified in the coding instructions, skip to the next item.

SOURCE: RAND

> **For the following questions, please consider only treatment provided to adult patients, including service members and family members, that [WEB: is][TELEPHONE: you] delivered at a military treatment facility including outpatient primary or specialty care clinics or "aid station" style settings.**
>
> *[Show PC1-PC3 on a single screen. Show PC4-PC6 on a second screen (with the same instructions repeated]*

PC1: What percent of your current patients have a PTSD diagnosis? [**Telephone:** Would you say...]	○ None *[If checked, skip to PC4]* ○ 1-25% ○ 26-50% ○ More than 50% *[If respondent declines to answer, skip to PC4]*
PC2: Please estimate the average number of visits that you see a patient with PTSD in a typical course of treatment. [**Telephone:** Would you say you see them for...]	○ 1 to 3 ○ 4 to 7 ○ 8 to 12 ○ More than 12

PC3: Taking into account your current caseload, how often are you able to see a patient with PTSD? [**Telephone:** Would you say...]	○ Weekly or more often ○ Every two weeks ○ Every three weeks ○ Monthly ○ Less than monthly
PC4: What percent of your current patients have a Major Depressive Disorder (or MDD) diagnosis? [**Telephone:** Would you say...]	○ None *[If checked, skip to PC7]* ○ 1-25% ○ 26-50% ○ More than 50% *[If respondent declines to answer, skip to PC7]*
PC5: Please estimate the average number of visits that you see a patient with MDD in a typical course of treatment. [**Telephone:** Would you say you see them...]	○ 1 to 3 ○ 4 to 7 ○ 8 to 12 ○ More than 12
PC6: Taking into account your current caseload, how often are you able to see a patient with MDD? [**Telephone:** Would you say...]	○ Weekly or more often ○ Every two weeks ○ Every three weeks ○ Monthly ○ Less than monthly
Now considering ALL of the patients that you see at a military treatment facility, including both adults and children, *[Show instructions and items PC7-PC8 on single screen]*	
PC7: Please estimate the average number of patient visits that you complete in a typical week. (Count visits where multiple patients were seen, as in group or couples therapy, as one visit.) [TELEPHONE: ONLY DISPLAY THIS...] [PROMPT IF RESPONDENT PROVIDES A RANGE: If you had to give an average number of visits within that range, what would you say?]	_____ visits (0–200) [If PC7=0, skip to PC9] *[If respondent declines to answer, skip to PC9]*

PC8: Typically, how many of these visits are completed in a *primary care setting*?	___ of the *[populate PC7 response]* visits are completed in a *primary care setting*. (Enter zero if you do not see any patients in a primary care setting.)

Theoretical Orientation

[WEB VERSION]
PC9. Place a one (1) next to your primary theoretical orientation and a two (2) next to your secondary theoretical orientation? **[SOURCE: Norcross & Rogan, 2013]**

[TELEPHONE VERSION]
From the following list that I will read, please tell me your primary theoretical orientation. Is it …

[READ LIST AND PLACE "1" BY PRIMARY ORIENTATION.]

What is your secondary theoretical orientation?
[INTERVIEWER: If no secondary orientation, just leave that blank and continue.]

[PLACE "2" BY SECONDARY ORIENTATION. ONLY READ LIST A SECOND TIME IF REQUESTED]

[INTERVIEWER: If the respondent states cognitive/behavioral, say: "I have an option for cognitive and a separate option for behavioral. Can you tell me which one you would consider your primary orientation and which one is secondary?"]

___ Acceptance / Third Wave
___ Behavioral
___ Biological
___ Cognitive
___ Existential
___ Experiential / Gestalt
___ Humanistic
___ Integrative / Eclectic
___ Interpersonal (IPT)
___ Psychoanalytic

___ Psychodynamic/Relational
___ Rogerian/Person-Centered
___ Systems/Family Systems
___ Other #1 (Please specify): _____
___ Other #2 (Please specify): _____

Measurement-Based Care

[WEB] How often do you or your clinic / practice setting support staff: [TELEPHONE] The following questions ask how often you or your clinic or practice setting support staff do a variety of things. Please answer "never" "seldom" "occasionally" "often" or "always" [PROMPT IF NECESSARY: Would you say "never" "seldom" "occasionally" "often" or "always"]	Never	Seldom	Occasionally	Often	Always
MBC1. [PHONE: How often do you or your support staff] Screen new patients for MDD using a validated screening instrument (for example the PHQ-2 or Patient Health Questionnaire)?	○	○	○	○	○
MBC2. [PHONE: How often do you or your support staff] Screen new patients for PTSD using a validated screening instrument (for example the PCL or PTSD Checklist)?	○	○	○	○	○
MBC3. [PHONE: How often do you or your support staff] Use a validated instrument of patient symptoms to inform adjustments in the patient's treatment plan?	○	○	○	○	○

Medication Management: Screening Items

MM1. <u>In the last 30 days</u>, did you prescribe a medication or have a medication management visit with an adult patient with <u>PTSD</u>?

     ○ No
     ○ Yes

MM2. <u>In the last 30 days</u>, did you prescribe a medication or have a medication management visit with a patient with <u>Major Depressive Disorder (or MDD)</u>?
     ○ No
     ○ Yes

Medication Management for PTSD

PURPOSE: PTSD provider behavior scale for prescribers

SOURCE: Adapted from Wilk J, West J, Duffy F, Herrell R, Rae D, Hoge C. (2013). Use of Evidence-Based Treatment for Posttraumatic Stress Disorder in Army Behavioral Health-care. *Psychiatry*; 76(4), 336-348

[WEB VERSION]

The next items will ask you about your <u>medication management</u> of an <u>adult patient with PTSD</u>.

Programming Note: If MM1='Yes', then continue.
If (MM1=('No' or respondent skipped) AND MM2='Yes), then skip to MM7.
If (MM1=('No' or respondent skipped) AND MM2=('No' or respondent skipped), then skip to PT1.

To select that patient, please open your charting or scheduling system (e.g., AHLTA, ESSEN-TRIS) to view your recent appointments. Please select the <u>most recent</u> adult patient with PTSD who you saw for a medication management visit.

If this visit was <u>more than 30 days ago</u>, **please check here ☐**. *[If checked AND MM2=yes, skip to MM7, else skip to PT1].*

If you do not currently have access to your charting or scheduling system (e.g., AHLTA, ESSENTRIS), **please check here ☐**. Please do your best to recall your most recent PTSD patient as you respond to these items.

[TELEPHONE VERSION]

The next questions will ask you about your medication management of an adult patient with PTSD.

To select that patient, please open your charting or scheduling system to view your recent appointments. Please select the most recent adult patient with PTSD who you saw for a medication management visit.

[PROMPT IF NECESSARY: Common charting systems include AHLTA (SAY: ALL-TA) for outpatient care and ESSENTRIS for inpatient care]

[Pause until respondent indicates they are ready]

[If respondent does not currently have access to his or her charting or scheduling system, check here ☐

And say:]

That's ok. Please do your best to recall your most recent PTSD patient as you respond to these items.

How long ago was the last visit? If the visit was <u>more than 30 days ago</u>, check here ☐
And say:]

Since it's been over a month since you saw them last, I need to skip to the next survey section.

To protect their privacy, please do not tell me the first or last name of this person. However, so that we can refer back to this same patient in case the interview is interrupted, please tell me the initial of the person's first name. For example, if the person's name is John, say 'J'. The patient's initial will be deleted from our files upon completion of the interview.

Patient initial: ___

[WEB] MM3. Considering your most recent patient with PTSD, in addition to PTSD, what other psychiatric diagnoses does this patient have? *(Please select all that apply)* **[TELEPHONE]** During the remainder of the interview I will refer to this person as patient <INSERT INITIAL> In addition to PTSD, does patient < > have any of the following diagnoses:	□ Adjustment disorder □ Anxiety disorder (other than PTSD) □ Depressive disorder □ Personality disorder □ Substance use disorder □ Relational problems (V-code) □ Other psychiatric diagnoses. Please specify:__ □ No other psychiatric diagnoses
[WEB] MM4. Does this patient's current prescriptions include psychopharmacologic medication? **[TELEPHONE]** MM4. Does patient < > current prescriptions include psychopharmacologic medication?	○ No ○ Yes ○ Don't know Programming Note: • If MM4='Yes', continue. • Else If ((MM4='No' or 'Don't Know' or respondent skipped) AND (MM2='Yes)), then skip to MM7. • Else If ((MM4='No' or Don't Know or respondent skipped) AND MM2=('No' or respondent skipped), then skip to PT1.

[WEB] **MM5. Scheduled Daily or Depot Psychopharmacologic Medications:** Provide the total dosage per day, not the administration instruction. If variable doses are used, provide a best estimate of average daily dose. For example, if fluoxetine is prescribed 20 mg qod, list as fluoxetine 10 mg/day; if fluoxetine is prescribed 10 mg/day and 20 mg/day on alternate days, list as 15 mg/day. Do not include PRN (as needed) medications. **[TELEPHONE]** MM5. I will ask about PRN **[as needed]** medications later, but first, please tell me the scheduled daily psychopharmacologic medications prescribed for this patient. Please tell me the medication name and total dosage per day. If variable doses are used, please tell me your best estimate of <u>average daily dose</u>. **[Respondent provides answer]** Next, please tell me the scheduled depot psychopharmacologic medications prescribed for this patient. Please tell me the medication names only. **[Respondent provides answer]** **[IF RESPONDENT IS CONFUSED, INTERVIEWER MAY SAY: For example, if fluoxetine is prescribed 20 mg qod, say fluoxetine 10 mg/day; if fluoxetine is prescribed 10 mg/day and 20 mg/day on alternate days, say 15 mg/day.]**	Current Total **Scheduled Daily**: Medication Name (Generic or Brand Name) _____ Current Total Dose Per Day: _____ mg/day [Space for 8 medications] ☐ No daily medications Current Total **Scheduled Depot** per Month Medication Name (Generic or Brand Name) _____ [Space for 2 depot medications] ☐ No depot medications

| [WEB]
MM6. **PRN** (as needed) **Psychopharmacologic Medications:** Please indicate total current maximum daily dose.

[TELEPHONE]
MM6 Finally, what PRN [**as needed**] psychopharmacologic medications are prescribed for this patient? Please tell me the medication name and the total current <u>maximum daily dose</u>. | Medication Name (Generic or Brand Name) _____

Current Total Dose Per Day: _____ mg/day
[Space for 5 medications]

☐ No PRN medications |

Programming Note: If MM2='Yes', then continue.

If MM2=('No' or respondent skipped), then skip to PT1.

Medication Management for MDD

PURPOSE: MDD provider behavior scale for prescribers

SOURCE: Adapted from Wilk J, West J, Duffy F, Herrell R, Rae D, Hoge C. (2013). Use of Evidence-Based Treatment for Posttraumatic Stress Disorder in Army Behavioral Healthcare. *Psychiatry*; 76(4), 336-348

[WEB]
The following questions will ask you about your <u>medication management</u> of an <u>adult patient with MDD</u>.

To select that patient, please open your charting or scheduling system (e.g., AHLTA, ESSEN-TRIS) to view your recent appointments. Please select the <u>most recent</u> adult patient with MDD who you saw for a medication management visit.

If this visit was <u>more than 30 days ago</u>, **please check here** ☐. *[If checked skip to PT1].*

If you do not currently have access to your charting or scheduling system (e.g., AHLTA, ESSENTRIS), **please check here** ☐. Please do you best to recall your most recent MDD patient as you respond to these items.

[TELEPHONE]

The following questions ask you about your <u>medication management</u> of an <u>adult patient with MDD</u>.

To select that patient, please open your charting or scheduling system to view your recent appointments. Please select the <u>most recent</u> adult patient with MDD who you saw for a medication management visit.

[PROMPT IF NECESSARY: Common charting systems include AHLTA (SAY: ALL-TA) and ESSENTRIS]

[Pause until respondent indicates they are ready]

[If respondent does not currently have access to his or her charting or scheduling system, check here ☐

And say:]

That's ok. Please do your best to recall your most recent MDD patient as you respond to these items.

How long ago was the last visit? If the visit was <u>more than 30 days ago</u>, check here ☐
And say:]

Since it's been over a month since you saw them last, I need to skip to the next survey section.

To protect their privacy, please do not tell me the first or last name of this person. However, so that we can refer back to this same patient in case the interview is interrupted, please tell me the initial of the person's first name. For example, if the person's name is John, say 'J'. The patient's initial will be deleted from our files upon completion of the interview.

Patient initial: _____

INTERVIEWER: If the respondent asks if it matters if this patient is the same as or different from the first patient, say: "No, as long as the person is your **most recent patient with MDD**, then it doesn't matter whether it's the same or different person from the last patient we included."

[WEB] MM7. Considering your most recent patient with MDD, in addition to MDD, what other psychiatric diagnoses does this patient have? *(Please select all that apply)* **[TELEPHONE]** MM7. During the remainder of the interview I will refer to this person as patient < >. In addition to MDD, does patient < > have any of the following diagnoses:	☐ Adjustment disorder ☐ Anxiety disorder (other than PTSD) ☐ PTSD ☐ Personality disorder ☐ Substance use disorder ☐ Relational problems (V-code) ☐ Other psychiatric diagnoses. Please specify: __ ☐ No other psychiatric diagnoses
[WEB] MM8. Does this patient's current prescriptions include psychopharmacologic medication? **[TELEPHONE]** MM8. Does patient < >'s current prescriptions include psychopharmacologic medication?	○ No ○ Yes ○ Don't know **Programming Note:** • If MM8='Yes', then continue. • Else If ((MM8='No' or 'Don't Know' or respondent skipped), skip to PT1.

[WEB] **MM9. Scheduled Daily or Depot Psychopharmacologic Medications:** Provide the total dosage per day, not the administration instruction. If variable doses are used, provide a best estimate of average daily dose. For example, if fluoxetine is prescribed 20 mg qod, list as fluoxetine 10 mg/day; if fluoxetine is prescribed 10 mg/day and 20 mg/day on alternate days, list as 15 mg/day. Do not include PRN (as needed) medications. **[TELEPHONE]** MM9. I will ask about PRN [**as needed**] medications later, but first, please tell me the scheduled daily psychopharmacologic medications prescribed for this patient. Please tell me the medication name and total dosage per day. If variable doses are used, please tell me your best estimate of <u>average daily dose</u>. [**Respondent provides answer**] Next, please tell me the scheduled depot psychopharmacologic medications prescribed for this patient. Please tell me the medication names only. [**Respondent provides answer**] **[IF RESPONDENT IS CONFUSED, INTERVIEWER MAY SAY: For example, if fluoxetine is prescribed 20 mg qod, list as fluoxetine 10 mg/day; if fluoxetine is prescribed 10 mg/day and 20 mg/day on alternate days, list as 15 mg/day.]**	Current Total <u>**Scheduled Daily**</u> Medication Name (Generic or Brand Name) _____ Current Total Dose Per Day: _____ mg/day *[Space for 8 medications]* ☐ No daily medications Current Total <u>**Scheduled Depot**</u> per Month Medication Name (Generic or Brand Name) _____ *[Space for 2 depot medications]* ☐ No depot medications
[WEB] MM10. **PRN** (as needed) **Psychopharmacologic Medications:** Please indicate total current maximum daily dose. **[TELEPHONE]** MM10. Finally, what PRN [**as needed**] psychopharmacologic medications are prescribed for this patient? Please tell me the medication name and the total current <u>maximum daily dose</u>.	Medication Name (Generic or Brand Name) _____ Current Total Dose Per Day: _____ mg/day *[Space for 5 medications]* ☐ No PRN medications

Psychotherapy/Psychological Counseling: Screening Items

[WEB]
Recall that the following questions pertain only to visits occurring in a military treatment facility (including military primary care or 'aid station' style settings).

[TELEPHONE]
The following questions pertain only to visits occurring in a military treatment facility which includes military primary care or 'aid station' style settings.

PT1. <u>In the last 30 days,</u> did you have a <u>psychological counseling or psychotherapy</u> visit with a patient with <u>PTSD</u>?
    ○ Yes
    ○ No

PT2. <u>In the last 30 days,</u> did you have a <u>psychological counseling or psychotherapy</u> visit with a patient with <u>Major Depressive Disorder (or MDD)</u>?
    ○ Yes
    ○ No

Programming Note: If (PT1=('No' or respondent skipped) AND PT2=('No' or respondent skipped), then skip to T1.
    If (PT1=(('No' or respondent skipped) AND PT2='Yes'), then skip to MDD1.
    Else continue.

Treatment Approaches for PTSD

[WEB] PTSD1. **Of the following treatment approaches, what types of therapy have you used to treat patients with PTSD?** *(Please select all that apply.)* **[TELEPHONE]** PTSD1. **Of the following treatment approaches that I will read, what types of therapy have you used to treat patients with <u>PTSD</u>? Have you used…?**	**[WEB]** PTSD2. **Of the therapies that you have used to treat patients with PTSD, what is the primary mode of therapy that you use to treat patients with PTSD?** *(Please select one primary treatment type.)* [Program to auto-respond to PTSD2 if only one therapy is selected for PTSD1] **[TELEPHONE]** PTSD2. **Of the therapies that you have used to treat patients with PTSD, what is the primary mode of therapy that you use to treat patients with PTSD?** [Interviewer may read populated list if needed]

☐ Acceptance and Commitment Therapy (ACT)	○ *[Populated from responses to PTSD1]*
☐ Behavioral Therapy / Behavioral Activation (BT/BA)	○ *[Populated from responses to PTSD1]*
☐ Brain stimulation (e.g., electroconvulsive therapy (ECT), transcranial magnetic stimulation	○ *[Populated from responses to PTSD1]*
☐ Cognitive Therapy	○ *[Populated from responses to PTSD1]*
☐ Cognitive Behavioral Therapy (CBT)	○ *[Populated from responses to PTSD1]*
☐ Cognitive Processing Therapy (CPT)	
☐ Complementary and alternative medicine (e.g., meditation, acupuncture)	
☐ Couples Therapy	
☐ Dialectical behavioral therapy (DBT)	
☐ Existential	
☐ Experiential / Gestalt	
☐ Exposure Therapy or Prolonged Exposure (PE)	
☐ Eye movement desensitization and reprocessing (EMDR)	
☐ Humanistic Therapy	
☐ Hypnosis	
☐ Imagery Rehearsal Therapy (IRT)	
☐ Integrative / Eclectic	
☐ Interpersonal Therapy (IPT)	
☐ Motivational Interviewing (MI)	
☐ Problem-Solving Therapy (PST)	
☐ Psychoanalysis	
☐ Time Limited Psychodynamic (TLDP)	
☐ Traditional Psychodynamic	
☐ Reality Therapy	
☐ Rogerian or other client centered approach	
☐ Seeking Safety	
☐ Stress Inoculation Training (SIT)	
☐ Supportive Counseling	
☐ Systems or Family Systems Therapy	
☐ Other. [PHONE- Something else that I didn't say?]. Please specify: _____	
[If respondent declines to answer, skip to PTSD3]	

Psychotherapy for PTSD

PURPOSE: Session behavior scale used to assess adherence to PTSD CPG recommendations (PE, CPT, EMDR)

SOURCE: Adapted from Wilk J, West J, Duffy F, Herrell R, Rae D, Hoge C. (2013). Use of Evidence-Based Treatment for Posttraumatic Stress Disorder in Army Behavioral Healthcare. *Psychiatry*; 76(4), 336–348

NOTE: This scale has been modified from the original response options (yes/no) to those shown in order to be consistent with the MDD behavior scale on pages 17–18. It has also been modified to query therapist behaviors rather than patient behaviors—again to be consistent with the MDD scale. In addition, some language referring to specific worksheets was modified to increase generalizability.

[WEB]
The following items will ask you about <u>psychological counseling</u> that you provided to an <u>adult patient with PTSD</u>.

To select that patient, please open your charting or scheduling system (e.g., AHLTA, ESSENTRIS) to view your recent appointments. Please select the <u>most recent</u> adult patient with PTSD with whom you had a <u>psychological counseling</u> visit.

If this visit was <u>more than 30 days ago</u>, **please check here** ☐. [If checked AND PT2=yes, skip to MDD1, else skip to T1].

If you do not currently have access to your charting or scheduling system (e.g., AHLTA, ESSENTRIS), **please check here** ☐. Please do your best to recall your most recent PTSD patient as you respond to these items.

[TELEPHONE]

The following items will ask you about psychological counseling that you provided to an adult patient with PTSD.

To select that patient, please open your charting or scheduling system to view your recent appointments. Please select the most recent adult patient with PTSD with whom you had a psychological counseling visit.

[PROMPT IF NECESSARY: Common charting systems include AHLTA (SAY: ALL-TA) and ESSENTRIS]

[Pause until respondent indicates they are ready].

[If respondent does not currently have access to his or her charting or scheduling system, check here ☐

And say:]

That's ok. Please do your best to recall your most recent PTSD patient as you respond to these items.

To protect their privacy, please do not tell me the first or last name of this person. However, so that we can refer back to this same patient in case the interview is interrupted, please tell me the initial of the person's first name. For example, if the person's name is John, say 'J'. The patient's initial will be deleted from our files upon completion of the interview.

Patient initial: _____

INTERVIEWER: If the respondent asks if it matters if this patient is the same as or different from the first patient, say: "No, as long as the person is your most recent patient with PTSD, then it doesn't matter whether it's the same or different person from the last patient we included."

How long ago was the last visit? If the visit was <u>more than 30 days ago</u>, check here ☐

And say:]

Since it's been over a month since you saw them last, I need to skip to the next survey section.

[WEB] PTSD3. Considering your most recent patient with PTSD, in addition to PTSD, what other psychiatric diagnoses does this patient have? *(Please select all that apply)* **[TELEPHONE]** PTSD3. During the remainder of the interview I will refer to this person as patient < >. In addition to PTSD, does patient < > have any of the following diagnoses:	☐ Adjustment disorder ☐ Anxiety disorder (other than PTSD) ☐ Depressive disorder ☐ Personality disorder ☐ Substance use disorder ☐ Relational problems (V-code) ☐ Other psychiatric diagnoses. Please specify: _____ ☐ No other psychiatric diagnoses
[WEB] PTSD4. How many visits have you had with this patient? **[TELEPHONE]** PTSD4. How many visits have you had with patient < >? **[PROMPT IF RESPONDENT PROVIDES A RANGE:** **If you had to give one number within that range, what would you say?]**	_____ visits

[WEB] In thinking of your sessions with this patient, HOW OFTEN: [TELEPHONE] In thinking of your sessions with patient < >, [PROMPT IF NECESSARY: Would you say "never" "almost never" "sometimes" "usually" "almost always" or "always"]	Never	Almost Never	Sometimes	Usually
PTSD5. How often, did you help this patient to identify the worst part of his/her trauma(s) and any negative associated cognitions?	O	O	O	O
PTSD6. How often, did you ask this patient to recount the traumatic event(s) aloud repeatedly, including telling you the details of the event, their thoughts and feelings? [IF PTSD6=('never' OR respondent skipped), then skip to PTSD7]	O	O	O	O
PTSD6a. How often, did this patient do this with their eyes closed?	O	O	O	O
PTSD6b. How often, did this patient recount the event in present tense?	O	O	O	O
PTSD7. How often, did you explore the deeper emotional meaning of this patient's concerns or behaviors (e.g., subconscious motives)?	O	O	O	O
PTSD8. How often, did you ask this patient to focus on the traumatic image, negative thoughts, and body sensations while moving his/her eyes back and forth to laterally track your finger?	O	O	O	O
PTSD9. How often, did you ask this patient to focus on the traumatic image, negative thoughts, and body sensations while tracking other auditory tones, tapping or other tactile stimulations?	O	O	O	O
PTSD10.How often, did you encourage this patient [PHONE: patient < >] to write about the meaning of his or her traumatic event as well as beliefs about why the event happened? [IF PTSD10=('never' OR respondent skipped) then skip to PTSD11]	O	O	O	O
PTSD10a. How often, did you ask this patient to read what they wrote out loud to you?	O	O	O	O

	Never	Almost Never	Sometimes	Usually
PTSD11. How often, did you assign self-monitoring homework to identify the connection between events, thoughts, and feelings?	○	○	○	○
PTSD12. How often, did you encourage this patient to think of a preferred positive belief to replace negative beliefs associated with his/her trauma?	○	○	○	○
PTSD13. How often, did you ask this patient to listen to a recording of his or her recounting of the traumatic event at home?	○	○	○	○
PTSD14. How often, did you encourage this patient to challenge and modify maladaptive thoughts and beliefs related to their traumatic experience?	○	○	○	○
PTSD15. How often, did you ask this patient to practice breathing and relaxation exercises at home?	○	○	○	○
PTSD16. How often, did you encourage this patient to challenge his or her over-generalized beliefs related to safety, trust, power/control, esteem, and intimacy?	○	○	○	○
PTSD17. How often, did you encourage this patient to talk about issues as they came to mind?	○	○	○	○
PTSD18. How often, did you assign in vivo (real-life) exposure tasks between sessions?	○	○	○	○

Programming Note: If PT2=yes, then continue.
     If PT2=('no' or respondent skipped), then skip to T1.

Treatment Approaches for MDD

[WEB] MDD1. **Of the following treatment approaches, what types of therapy have you used to treat patients with <u>MDD</u>?** *(Please select all that apply.)* **[TELEPHONE]** MDD1. **Of the following treatment approaches, what types of therapy have you used to treat patients with <u>MDD</u>? Have you used…?**	**[WEB]** MDD2. **Of the therapies that you have used to treat patients with MDD, what is the primary mode of therapy that you use to treat patients with MDD?** *(Please select one primary treatment type.)* [Program to auto-respond to MDD2 if only one therapy is selected for MDD1] **[TELEPHONE]** MDD2. **Of the therapies that you have used to treat patients with MDD, what is the primary mode of therapy that you use to treat patients with MDD?** [Interviewer may read populated list if needed]

□ Acceptance and Commitment Therapy (ACT)	○ [Populated from responses to MDD1]
□ Behavioral Therapy / Behavioral Activation (BT/BA)	○ [Populated from responses to MDD1]
□ Brain stimulation (e.g., electroconvulsive therapy (ECT), transcranial magnetic stimulation)	○ [Populated from responses to MDD1] ○ [Populated from responses to MDD1] ○ [Populated from responses to MDD1]
□ Cognitive Therapy	
□ Cognitive Behavioral Therapy (CBT)	
□ Cognitive Processing Therapy (CPT)	
□ Complementary and alternative medicine (e.g., meditation, acupuncture)	
□ Couples Therapy	
□ Dialectical behavioral therapy (DBT)	
□ Existential	
□ Experiential / Gestalt	
□ Exposure Therapy or Prolonged Exposure (PE)	
□ Eye movement desensitization and reprocessing (EMDR)	
□ Humanistic Therapy	
□ Hypnosis	
□ Imagery Rehearsal Therapy (IRT)	
□ Integrative / Eclectic	
□ Interpersonal Therapy (IPT)	
□ Motivational Interviewing (MI)	
□ Problem-Solving Therapy (PST)	
□ Psychoanalysis	
□ Time Limited Psychodynamic (TLDP)	
□ Traditional Psychodynamic	
□ Reality Therapy	
□ Rogerian, client centered approach	
□ Seeking Safety	
□ Stress Inoculation Training (SIT)	
□ Supportive Counseling	
□ Systems or Family Systems Therapy	
□ Other. [PHONE- Something else that I didn't say?] Please specify: _____	
[If respondent declines to answer, skip to MDD3]	

Psychotherapy for MDD

SOURCE: Adapted from Hepner K, Azocar F, Greenwood G, Miranda J, Burnam M. (2010). Development of a Clinician Report Measure to Assess Psychotherapy for Depression in Usual Care Settings. *Administration and Policy in Mental Health*; 37(3).

PURPOSE: Session behavior scale used to assess adherence to MDD CPG recommendations (Items assess CBT and IPT, while Psychodynamic therapy items assess deviation from these therapies). Excludes CPG 1st line treatment Problem-Solving Therapy (because usually in primary care)

[WEB]

The following items will ask you about <u>psychological counseling</u> that you provided to an <u>adult patient with MDD</u>.

To select that patient, please open your charting or scheduling system (e.g., AHLTA, ESSENTRIS) to view your recent appointments. Please select the <u>most recent</u> adult patient with MDD with whom you had a <u>psychological counseling</u> visit.

If this visit was <u>more than 30 days ago</u>, **please check here** ☐. [If checked, skip to T1].

If you do not currently have access to your charting or scheduling system (e.g., AHLTA, ESSENTRIS), **please check here** ☐. Please do you best to recall your most recent patient with MDD as you respond to these items.

[TELEPHONE]

The following items will ask you about <u>psychological</u> counseling that you provided to an <u>adult patient with MDD</u>.

To select that patient, please open your charting or scheduling system to view your recent appointments. Please select the <u>most recent</u> adult patient with MDD with whom you had a <u>psychological counseling</u> visit.

[PROMPT IF NECESSARY: Common charting systems include AHLTA (SAY: ALL-TA) and ESSENTRIS]

[Pause until respondent indicates they are ready]

[If respondent does not currently have access to his or her charting or scheduling system, check here ☐

And say:]

That's ok. Please do your best to recall your most recent MDD patient as you respond to these items.

How long ago was the last visit? If the visit was <u>more than 30 days ago</u>, check here ☐

And say:]

Since it's been over a month since you saw them last, I need to skip to the next survey section.

To protect their privacy, please do not tell me the first or last name of this person. However, so that we can refer back to this same patient in case the interview is interrupted, please tell me the initial of the person's first name. For example, if the person's name is John, say 'J'. The patient's initial will be deleted from our files upon completion of the interview.

Patient initial: _____

INTERVIEWER: If the respondent asks if it matters if this patient is the same as or different from the first patient, say: "No, as long as the person is your most recent patient with MDD, then it doesn't matter whether it's the same or different person from the last patient we included."

[WEB] MDD3. Considering your most recent patient with MDD, in addition to MDD, what other psychiatric diagnoses does this patient have? *(Please select all that apply)* **[TELEPHONE]** MDD3. During the remainder of the inter-view I will refer to this person as patient < >. In addition to MDD, does patient < > have any of the fol-lowing diagnoses:	□ Adjustment disorder □ Anxiety disorder (other than PTSD) □ PTSD □ Personality disorder □ Substance use disorder □ Relational problems (V-code) □ Other psychiatric diag-noses. Please specify: _____ □ No other psychiatric diagnoses
[WEB] MDD4. How many visits have you had with this patient? **[TELEPHONE]** How many visits have you had with patient < >? **[PROMPT IF RESPONDENT PROVIDES A RANGE: If you had to give one number within that range, what would you say?]**	_____ visits

[WEB] In thinking of your sessions with this patient, HOW OFTEN: [TELEPHONE] The following questions ask how often you used a variety of clinical techniques with patient F. Please answer each question with "never" "almost never" "sometimes" "usually" "almost always" or "always" In thinking of your sessions with this patient, HOW OFTEN…	Never	Almost Never	Sometimes	Usually	Almost Always	Always	[Sub-scale]
MDD5. How often, did you discuss the current quality of patient's relationships with other people?	○	○	○	○	○	○	[IPT]
MDD6. How often, did you help this patient understand which thoughts are helpful and which thoughts are not (e.g. explain the cognitive triad, identify negative thinking)?	○	○	○	○	○	○	[CBT]
MDD7. How often, did you examine the emotional response the patient had during interpersonal interactions?	○	○	○	○	○	○	[IPT]
MDD8. How often, did you help this patient create statements they could use to respond to negative thoughts (e.g. practicing rational responses, using reattribution or alternative reasoning)?	○	○	○	○	○	○	[CBT]
MDD9. How often, did you encourage this patient to talk about issues as they came to mind?	○	○	○	○	○	○	[Dynamic]
MDD10. How often, did you assign "homework" between sessions (e.g. asked patient to complete Mood Rating Scale or a record of thoughts, feelings, or activities)?	○	○	○	○	○	○	[CBT]
MDD11. How often, did you help this patient to understand that addressing interpersonal situations may help improve their MDD?	○	○	○	○	○	○	[IPT]
MDD12. How often, did you ask this patient to do things they enjoyed doing between sessions (e.g. behavioral activation, increasing pleasurable activities, use of pleasure ratings)?	○	○	○	○	○	○	[CBT]
MDD13. How often, did you assess the positive and negative aspects of how this patient got along with others in the past (i.e. a prior social role, dysfunctional patterns, depth of intimacy in previous relationships?	○	○	○	○	○	○	[IPT]
MDD14. How often, did you explore the deeper emotional meaning of this patient's concerns or behaviors (e.g., subconscious motives)?	○	○	○	○	○	○	[Dynamic]
MDD15. How often, did you help this patient understand the beliefs and assumptions behind their thinking (e.g. core beliefs, cognitive schemas?	○	○	○	○	○	○	[CBT]

Training, Supervision and Confidence in PTSD and MDD Treatment Approaches

	Treatments for PTSD					Treatments for MDD			
	Medication Management for PTSD	Prolonged Exposure for PTSD	Cognitive Processing Therapy for PTSD	Eye Movement Desensitization and Reprocessing for PTSD	Stress Inoculation Training for PTSD	Medication Management for MDD	Interpersonal Therapy (IPT) for MDD	Cognitive Behavioral Therapy (CBT) for MDD	Problem-Solving Therapy for MDD
T1. **[BOTH WEB AND TELEPHONE]** The next questions ask about any formal training you have received in a variety of treatment approaches. <u>Formal training</u> refers to instruction delivered by an instructor in a class, workshop, lecture series, seminar, or webinar. Please do <u>not</u> include self-directed learning such as time reading journals, books, or websites. Approximately how many hours of <u>formal training</u> have you ever received in the following treatment approaches: [SOURCE: Wilk J, West J, Duffy F, Herrell R, Rae D, Hoge C. (2013). Use of Evidence-Based Treatment for Posttraumatic Stress Disorder in Army Behavioral Healthcare. *Psychiatry*;76(4), 336-348]	___ None ___ 1 to 8 hours ___ More than 8 hours	"	"	"	"	"	"	"	"

	Treatments for <u>PTSD</u>					Treatments for <u>MDD</u>			
	Medication Management for PTSD	Prolonged Exposure for PTSD	Cognitive Processing Therapy for PTSD	Eye Movement Desensitization and Reprocessing for PTSD	Stress Inoculation Training for PTSD	Medication Management for MDD	Interpersonal Therapy (IPT) for MDD	Cognitive Behavioral Therapy (CBT) for MDD	Problem-Solving Therapy for MDD
T2. **[BOTH WEB AND TELEPHONE]** The next questions ask about any <u>direct supervision or consultation</u> you have received in a variety of treatment approaches._ <u>Direct supervision or consultation</u> refers to supervision clinicians receive from an expert clinician when initially applying a treatment approach. Supervision of cases is typically beyond the training received during a workshop or class. Count only the hours you spent with your supervisor (by phone or in person). Note that supervision or consultation hours can occur while still in a training program or after beginning a professional career. How many hours of <u>direct supervision or consultation</u> have you ever received in the following treatment approaches: [SOURCE: RAND]	___ None ___ 1 to 8 hours ___ 9 to 20 hours ___ More than 20 hours	"	"	"	"	"	"	"	"

	Treatments for <u>PTSD</u>					Treatments for <u>MDD</u>			
	Medication Management for PTSD	Prolonged Exposure for PTSD	Cognitive Processing Therapy for PTSD	Eye Movement Desensitization and Reprocessing for PTSD	Stress Inoculation Training for PTSD	Medication Management for MDD	Interpersonal Therapy (IPT) for MDD	Cognitive Behavioral Therapy (CBT) for MDD	Problem–Solving Therapy for MDD
[WEB] T3. How confident are you in your ability to deliver each of the following treatment approaches: **[TELEPHONE]** How confident are you in your ability to deliver each of the following treatment approaches: Please answer "not at all confident" "somewhat confident" "moderately confident" or "very confident"	○ Not at all confident ○ Somewhat confident ○ Moderately confident ○ Very Confident	"	"	"	"	"	"	"	"

Barriers to Implementing CPG Recommended Care

Source: RAND developed these items following a review of existing measures and reports (Aarons et al., 2012; American Psychiatric Association (APA), 1996; Borah, 2013; Center for Deployment Psychology, 2013; Maslach et al., 1996; Meredith et al., 1999). Source information is noted on those items that are from or adapted from existing measures.

NOTE: Items are currently grouped by domain for ease of review, but were shuffled for the final survey.

[WEB] Please indicate your level of agreement with the following statements about treatment for patients with PTSD or MDD. [TELEPHONE] Next, I will read a series of statements about treatment for patients with PTSD or MDD. Please indicate your level of agreement by saying "strongly disagree", "disagree", "neither disagree nor agree", "agree" or "strongly agree". [PROMPT IF NECESSARY: Would you say you "strongly disagree", "disagree", "neither disagree nor agree", "agree" or "strongly agree".]	Strongly Disagree	Disagree	Neither Disagree nor Agree	Agree	Strongly Agree	[Level]	[Domain]
B1. Therapies that work well in a research setting don't work well with real patients.	○	○	○	○	○	[Provider]	[Attitudes toward research]
B2. If I am uncertain how to treat a patient, I consult with a trusted colleague or an expert clinician.	○	○	○	○	○	[Provider]	[Attitudes toward research]
B3. Clinical practice guidelines do not provide useful guidance for treating individual patients. [SOURCE: Adapted from APA, 1997]	○	○	○	○	○	[Provider]	[Attitudes toward standardized practice]
B4. Clinical experience is more important than the recommendations of clinical practice guidelines. [SOURCE: Adapted from Aarons et al. (2012)]	○	○	○	○	○	[Provider]	[Attitudes toward standardized practice]

	Strongly Disagree	Disagree	Neither Disagree nor Agree	Agree	Strongly Agree	[Level]	[Domain]
B5. Structured, manualized treatment approaches are boring for an experienced therapist. [SOURCE: Adapted from Center for Deployment Psychology (2013) recommendations]	o	o	o	o	o	[Provider]	[Attitudes toward standardized practice]
B6. I am able to treat my patients according to my own best judgment. [SOURCE: Adapted Meredith et al. (1999)]	o	o	o	o	o	[Facility]	[Autonomy vs accountability]
B7. Leadership expects me to deliver a certain kind of treatment/therapy to my patients.	o	o	o	o	o	[Facility]	[Autonomy vs accountability]
B8. I don't have the time in my schedule to see patients as often as I would like.	o	o	o	o	o	[Facility]	[Caseload/workload]
B9. I am so busy that I don't have time to learn a new therapy. [SOURCE: Adapted from Center for Deployment Psychology (2013) recommendations]	o	o	o	o	o	[Facility]	[Caseload/workload]
B10. I feel emotionally drained from my work. [SOURCE: Maslach et al., 1996]	o	o	o	o	o	[Facility/Provider]	[Burnout]
B11. I feel I'm positively influencing my patients lives through my work. [SOURCE: Maslach et al., 1996]	o	o	o	o	o	[Facility/Provider]	[Burnout]
B12. Research has shown that all therapies are about equally effective.	o	o	o	o	o	[Provider]	[Dodo bird]
B13. Nonspecific aspects of therapy, like good rapport, are the best predictors of treatment success.	o	o	o	o	o	[Provider]	[Dodo bird]

	Strongly Disagree	Disagree	Neither Disagree nor Agree	Agree	Strongly Agree	[Level]	[Domain]
B14. My patients' military duties limit their ability to receive appropriate care (e.g., patient PCS, deployment, irregular work schedules).	○	○	○	○	○	[Patient]	[Military specific]
B15. Limitations on travel prevent me from receiving additional training.	○	○	○	○	○	[Facility]	[Military specific]
B16. If I learned a treatment was successful with patients like mine, I would make it a priority to learn the new treatment.	○	○	○	○	○	[Provider]	[Openness]
B17. Patient preferences influence my treatment approach. [SOURCE: Adapted from Borah (2013)]	○	○	○	○	○	[Patient]	[Patient-centered care]
B18. Manualized treatment approaches prevent therapists from responding to the unique needs of each patient. [SOURCE: Adapted from Center for Deployment Psychology (2013) recommendations]	○	○	○	○	○	[Provider]	[Patient-centered care]
B19. My supervisor supports ongoing professional training (e.g., hosts workshops, reimburses travel costs).	○	○	○	○	○	[Facility]	[Training/ supervision resources]
B20. I have protected time in my schedule to attend workshops/seminars to improve my clinical skills.	○	○	○	○	○	[Facility]	[Training supervision resources]
B21. Providers at my site have access to expert clinical supervisors.	○	○	○	○	○	[Facility]	[Training/ supervision resources]
B22. Patients' commanders defer to my clinical expertise with respect to patients' need for treatment and length of treatment.	○	○	○	○	○	[Provider]	[Command communication]

	Strongly Disagree	Disagree	Neither Disagree nor Agree	Agree	Strongly Agree	[Level]	[Domain]
B23. I am comfortable sharing information about my patients' psychological health and treatment course with their commanders as necessary.	○	○	○	○	○	[Provider]	[Command communication]
B24. I believe patients' commanders should be aware of the patients' need for treatment.	○	○	○	○	○	[Provider]	[Command communication]
B25. It is easy for me (or support staff at my site) to routinely track patient symptoms and response to treatment over time.	○	○	○	○	○	[Facility]	[Support for measurement-based care]
B26. I am well-supported by case managers (e.g., coordinating interdisciplinary care, follow-up with patients who do not attend appointments).	○	○	○	○	○	[Facility]	[Support for measurement-based care]

Provider Characteristics

[Source: RAND]

The final set of questions requests important background and demographic information that will help us to describe the group of respondents to this survey.

DEMO1: Are you a…	○ Clinical Psychologist (PhD or PsyD) ○ Licensed Clinical Social Worker (LCSW or MCSW) ○ Master's-Level, Licensed Professional Counselor (e.g., LPC or LMHC) ○ Psychiatrist (MD or DO) ○ Psychiatric Nurse Practitioner ○ Other (Please describe _____)
DEMO2: How many years have you practiced since earning your highest degree? **[TELEPHONE]** **[PROMPT IF RESPONDENT PROVIDES A RANGE: If you had to give one number within that range, what would you say?]**	_____ years
DEMO3: Are you of Hispanic or Latino origin or descent?	○ No ○ Yes
[WEB] DEMO4: What is your race? Please select one or more. **[TELEPHONE]** DEMO4: What is your race?	☐ White ☐ Black or African American ☐ Asian ☐ Native Hawaiian or Other Pacific Islander ☐ American Indian or Alaskan Native ☐ None of these (Please describe_____)
DEMO5: Please indicate your military status:	☐ Active Component ☐ National Guard ☐ Reserve ☐ DoD Civilian ☐ Other (Please describe _____)

DEMO6: What service branch do you work in?	☐ Army ☐ Navy ☐ Air Force ☐ Marines ☐ Other (Please describe _____)

[WEB]

Thank you for completing our survey. As a token of appreciation, we are able to send you a **$50** gift card via email if you completed this survey during off-duty time Which **$50** gift card would you like to receive?	☐ $50 Amazon gift card ☐ $50 Starbucks gift card ☐ $50 PayPal credit ☐ I would like to decline the gift card.
The gift card will come directly to your e-mail. What e-mail address should we send it to? We will only use that e-mail for the purposes of sending you the gift card.	E-mail address: _____ ☐ Prefer not to provide e-mail and forgo the gift card

[TELEPHONE]

Thank you for completing our survey. As a token of appreciation, we are able to send you a **$50** gift card via email if you completed this survey during off-duty time Which **$50** gift card would you like to receive?	☐ $50 Amazon gift card ☐ $50 Starbucks gift card ☐ $50 PayPal credit ☐ Respondent declined gift card
The gift card will come directly to your e-mail? What e-mail address should we send it to? We will only use that e-mail for the purposes of sending you the gift card.	E-mail address: _____ ☐ Prefer not to provide e-mail and forgo the gift card

Below are the patient initials collected during the interview, if any. Now that this interview is Complete or Termed, the initial will be deleted. Press next to delete: **Patient initial:** _r____ **Patient initial:** _y____ **Patient initial:** _m____ **Patient initial:** _x____	
This screen shows that all patient initials have been deleted: **Patient initial:** _____ **Patient initial:** _____ **Patient initial:** _____ **Patient initial:** _____	

[CLOSING/THANK YOU TEXT]

Thank you for taking the time to complete this survey. Your responses provide important insight into the experiences of military mental health providers and mental health treatment for service members.

Key Informant Interview Discussion Guide

What is your role with respect to the delivery of Behavioral Health Care in the MHS?

1. What are your specific responsibilities with respect to
   a. Workforce issues: Size, composition, scope of practice, training?
   b. BH Utilization and Performance management?
   c. Specific efforts (programs or policies) for improving quality of BH care?

2. Behavioral health workforce
   a. Can you give us an overview of the characteristics of the behavioral health workforce in terms of discipline, training background, capabilities, etc.?
   b. How are providers assigned, are they empaneled, are they able to specialize in specific treatments?
   c. How is provider performance assessed and/or monitored, etc.?
      ◦ What specific criteria or processes are used to determine if care is evidence based, appropriate or high quality?
      ◦ How is feedback provided to individual providers?

   d. What are the major workforce training initiatives for BH providers?
      ◦ Are there other sources of support, at the clinic or command level, for BH providers around EBT?
      ◦ How are ancillary mental health providers (chaplains, technicians, occupational therapists) engaged with the formal health system?

3. Utilization Management and Performance Measurement in Behavioral Health
   a. What are the major initiatives in this area?
      ◦ Who is responsible?
      ◦ How is it implemented?
         i. Have there been any major issues/challenges in rolling this out? If so, what are they and how are they being addressed?
         ii. What are the data sources used?
         iii. What is the reporting framework used?
         iv. Are there any standardized templates for data entry used, for example for managing behavioral health care?
         v. Have there been any major issues/challenges in rolling this out? If so, what are they and how are they being addressed?

    b. What are the incentives/disincentives involved in managing the delivery of behavioral health within ___?

4. Quality Improvement Efforts
    a. Are there any specific initiatives in place for improving quality of care?
    b. What are the major barriers and facilitators to improving access and quality within MHS?
    c. How is the quality of the system articulated within the system to patients, providers, and officials?

References

Aarons, Gregory A., Guy Cafri, Lindsay Lugo, and Angelina Sawitzky, "Expanding the Domains of Attitudes Towards Evidence-Based Practice: The Evidence Based Practice Attitude Scale—50," *Administration and Policy in Mental Health and Mental Health Services Research*, Vol. 39, No. 5, September 2012, pp. 331–340.

Academy of Cognitive Therapy, "ACT Certification," 2016. As of August 24, 2016:
http://www.academyofct.org/certification/

Acosta, Joie D., Amariah Becker, Jennifer L. Cerully, Michael P. Fisher, Laurie T. Martin, Raffaele Vardavas, Mary E. Slaugher, and Terry L. Schell, *Mental Health Stigma in the Military*, Santa Monica, Calif.: RAND Corporation, RR-426-OSD, 2014. As of August 16, 2016:
http://www.rand.org/pubs/research_reports/RR426.html

Air Force Medical Service, "Behavioral Health Optimization Program (BHOP)," 2013. As of January 6, 2017:
http://www.airforcemedicine.af.mil/About/Fact-Sheets/Display/Article/425489/
behavioral-health-optimization-program-bhop/

American Association for Public Opinion Research, "Response Rates—An Overview," undated. As of August 16, 2016:
http://www.aapor.org/Education-Resources/For-Researchers/Poll-Survey-FAQ/Response-Rates-An-Overview.aspx

American Psychiatric Association, *Improving Treatment for Depression: Survey of Participating Psychiatrists*, Arlington, Va., 1996.

———, *Practice Guideline for the Treatment of Patients with Acute Stress Disorder and Posttraumatic Stress Disorder*, Washington, D.C., 2004.

———, *Practice Guideline for the Treatment of Patients with Major Depressive Disorder*, Washington, D.C., 2010.

Batka, Caroline, Terri Tanielian, Mahlet A. Woldetsadik, Carrie Farmer, and Lisa Jaycox, "Stakeholder Experiences in a Stepped Collaborative Care Study Within U.S. Army Clinics," *Psychosomatics*, Vol. 57, No. 6, 2016, pp. 586–597.

Benedek, David M., Matthew J. Friedman, Douglas Zatzick, and Robert J. Ursano, "Guideline Watch (March 2009): Practice Guideline for the Treatment of Patients with Acute Stress Disorder and Posttraumatic Stress Disorder," *Focus*, Vol. 7, No. 2, Spring 2009, pp. 204–213.

Benjamini, Yoav, and Yosef Hochberg, "Controlling the False Discovery Rate: A Practical and Powerful Approach to Multiple Testing," *Journal of the Royal Statistical Society, Series B (Methodological)*, Vol. 57, No. 1, 1995, pp. 289–300.

Blakeley, Katherine, and Don J. Jansen, *Post-Traumatic Stress Disorder and Other Mental Health Problems in the Military: Oversight Issues for Congress*, Washington, D.C.: Congressional Research Service, 2013. As of October 5, 2015:
https://fas.org/sgp/crs/natsec/R43175.pdf

Borah, Elisa V., Edward C. Wright, D. Allen Donahue, Elizabeth M. Cedillos, David S. Riggs, William C. Isler, and Alan L. Peterson, "Implementation Outcomes of Military Provider Training in Cognitive Processing Therapy and Prolonged Exposure Therapy for Post-Traumatic Stress Disorder," *Military Medicine*, Vol. 178, No. 9, September 2013, pp. 939–944.

Brady, Kathleen, Teri Pearlstein, Gregory M. Asnis, Dewleen Baker, Barbara Rothbaum, Carolyn R. Sikes, and Gail M. Farfel, "Efficacy and Safety of Sertraline Treatment of Posttraumatic Stress Disorder: A Randomized Controlled Trial," *Journal of the American Medical Association*, Vol. 283, No. 14, April 12, 2000, pp. 1837–1844.

Burnette, Crystal, Rajeev Ramchand, and Lynsay Ayer, *Gatekeeper Training for Suicide Prevention: A Theoretical Model and Review of the Empirical Literature*, Santa Monica, Calif.: RAND Corporation, RR-1002-OSD, 2015. As of February 15, 2017:
http://www.rand.org/pubs/research_reports/RR1002.html

Center for Deployment Psychology, *Lessons Learned Manual: A Framework for Addressing Barriers to Evidence-Based Psychotherapy Utilization in the Defense Department*, Bethesda, Md.: Center for Deployment Psychology, 2013.

———, "CDP Training Opportunities," web page, undated. As of August 1, 2016:
http://deploymentpsych.org/psychological-training

Damschroder, Laura J., David C. Aron, Rosalind E. Keith, Susan R. Kirsh, Jeffery A. Alexander, and Julie C. Lowery, "Fostering Implementation of Health Services Research Findings into Practice: A Consolidated Framework for Advancing Implementation Science," *Implementation Science*, Vol. 4, No. 1, September 2009.

Davidson, Jonathan R., Barbara O. Rothbaum, Bessel A. van der Kolk, Carolyn R. Sikes, and Gail M. Farfel, "Multicenter, Double-Blind Comparison of Sertraline and Placebo in the Treatment of Posttraumatic Stress Disorder," *Archives of General Psychiatry*, Vol. 58, No. 5, May 2001, pp. 485–492.

Defense Centers of Excellence for Psychological Health & Traumatic Brain Injury, "Education Opportunites," 2016. As of October 31, 2016:
http://www.dcoe.mil/Training/Education.aspx

Defense Manpower Data Center, "Active Duty Military Strength by Service: Current Strength," 2016. As of January 10, 2017:
https://www.dmdc.osd.mil/appj/dwp/dwp_reports.jsp

Department of Defense, "Military Health System Review: Final Report to the Secretary of Defense," August 2014. As of August 15, 2016:
http://www.defense.gov/Portals/1/Documents/pubs/140930_MHS_Review_Final_Report_Main_Body.pdf

Department of Defense, Department of Veterans Affairs, Department of Health and Human Services, "Interagency Task Force on Military and Veterans Mental Health," 2013. As of October 31, 2016:
http://www.mentalhealth.va.gov/docs/2013_ITF_Report-FINAL.pdf

Department of Veterans Affairs and Department of Defense, "VA/DOD Clinical Practice Guideline for Management of Major Depressive Disorder. Version 3.0," 2016. As of May 27, 2016:
http://www.healthquality.va.gov/guidelines/mh/mdd/index.asp

Engel, Charles C., Lisa H. Jaycox, Michael C. Freed, Robert M. Bray, Donald Brambilla, Douglas F. Zatzick, Brett T. Litz, Terri Tanielian, Laura A. Novak, Marian E. Lane, Bradley E. Belsher, Kristine Rae Olmsted, Daniel P. Evatt, Russ Vandermaas-Peeler, Jurgen Unutzer, and Wayne J. Katon, "Centrally Assisted Collaborative Telecare for Posttraumatic Stress Disorder and Depression Among Military Personnel Attending Primary Care: A Randomized Clinical Trial," *JAMA: Internal Medicine*, Vol. 176, No. 7, 2016, pp. 948–956.

Erekson, David M., Michael J. Lambert, and Dennis L. Eggett, "The Relationship Between Session Frequency and Psychotherapy Outcome in a Naturalistic Setting," *Journal of Counsulting and Clinical Psychology*, Vol. 83, No. 6, December 2015, pp. 1097–1107.

Foa, Edna B., Jonathan R. T. Davidson, and Allen Frances, "The Expert Consensus Guideline Series: Treatment of Posttraumatic Stress Disorder," *Journal of Clinical Psychiatry*, Vol. 60, Suppl. 16, 1999, pp. 6–76.

Fulton, Jessica J., Patrick S. Calhoun, H. Ryan Wagner, Amie R. Schry, Lauren P. Hair, Nicole Feeling, Eric Elbogen, and Jean C. Beckham, "The Prevalence of Post-Traumatic Stress Disorder in Operation Enduring Freedom/Operation Iraqi Freedom (OEF/OIF) Veterans: A Meta-Analysis," *Journal of Anxiety Disorders*, Vol. 31, April 2015, pp. 98–107.

Harding, Kelli Jane, A. John Rush, Melissa Arbuckle, Madhukar H. Trivedi, and Harold Alan Pincus, "Measurement-Based Care in Psychiatric Practice: A Policy Framework for Implementation," *Journal of Clinical Psychiatry*, Vol. 72, No. 8, 2011, pp. 1136–1143.

Hawley, Kristin M., Jonathan R. Cook, and Amanda Jensen-Doss, "Do Noncontingent Incentives Increase Survey Response Rates Among Mental Health Providers? A Randomized Trial Comparison," *Administration and Policy in Mental Health and Mental Health Services Research*, Vol. 36, No. 5, September 2009, pp. 343–348.

Hepner, Kimberly A., Francisca Azocar, Gregory L. Greenwood, Jeanne Miranda, and M. Audrey Burnam, "Development of a Clinician Report Measure to Assess Psychotherapy for Depression in Usual Care Settings," *Administration and Policy in Mental Health and Mental Health Services Research*, Vol. 37, No. 3, May 2010, pp. 221–229.

Hepner, Kimberly A., Elizabeth M. Sloss, Carol P. Roth, Heather Krull, Susan M. Paddock, Shaela Moen, Martha J. Timmer, and Harold Alan Pincus, *Quality of Care for PTSD and Depression in the Military Health System: Phase 1 Report*, Santa Monica, Calif.: RAND Corporation, RR-978-OSD, 2016. As of August 19, 2016:
http://www.rand.org/pubs/research_reports/RR978.html

———, *Quality of Care for PTSD and Depression in the Military Health System: Final Report*, Santa Monica, Calif.: RAND Corporation, RR-1542-OSD, 2017.

Hoge, Charles W., Jennifer L. Auchterlonie, and Charles S. Milliken, "Mental Health Problems, Use of Mental Health Services, and Attrition from Military Service After Returning from Deployment to Iraq or Afghanistan," *JAMA*, Vol. 295, No. 9, March 1, 2006, pp. 1023–1032.

Hoge, Charles W., Carl A. Castro, Stephen C. Messer, Dennis McGurk, Dave I. Cotting, and Robert L. Koffman, "Combat Duty in Iraq and Afghanistan, Mental Health Problems, and Barriers to Care," *New England Journal of Medicine*, Vol. 351, July 1, 2004, pp. 13–22.

Hoge, Charles W., Christopher G. Ivany, Edward A. Brusher, Millard D. Brown III, John C. Shero, Amy B. Adler, Christopher H. Warner, and David T. Orman, "Transformation of Mental Health Care for U.S. Soldiers and Families During the Iraq and Afghanistan Wars: Where Science and Politics Intersect," *American Journal of Psychiatry*, Vol. 173, No. 4, April 1, 2015, pp. 334–343.

Institute of Medicine, *Treatment for Posttraumatic Stress Disorder in Military and Veteran Populations: Final Assessment*, Washington, D.C.: National Academies Press, 2014.

Jonas, Daniel E., Karen Cusack, Catherine A. Forneris, Tania M. Wilkins, Jeffrey Sonis, Jennifer Cook Middleton, Cynthia Feltner, Dane Meredith, Jamie Cavanaugh, Kimberly A. Brownley, Kristine Rae Olmsted, Amy Greenblatt, Amy Weil, and Bradley N. Gaynes, *Psychological and Pharmacological Treatments for Adults with Posttraumatic Stress Disorder (PTSD)*, Rockville, Md., Agency for Healthcare Research and Quality, Comparative Effectiveness Review No. 92, April 2013.

Kellerman, Scott E., and Joan Herold, "Physician Response to Surveys: A Review of the Literature," *American Journal of Preventive Medicine*, Vol. 20, No. 1, January 2001, pp. 61–67.

Levy, Claire M., Harry J. Thie, Jerry M. Sollinger, and Jennifer H. Kawata, *Army PERSTEMPO in the Post Cold War Era*, Santa Monica, Calif.: RAND Corporation, MR-1032-OSD, 2001. As of August 19, 2016:
http://www.rand.org/pubs/monograph_reports/MR1032.html

Maguen, Shira, Barbara A. Lucenko, Mark A. Reger, Gregory A. Gahm, Brett T. Litz, Karen H. Seal, Sara J. Knight, and Charles R. Marmar, "The Impact of Reported Direct and Indirect Killing on Mental Health Symptoms in Iraq War Veterans," *Journal of Traumatic Stress*, Vol. 23, No. 1, February 2010, pp. 86–90.

Management of Major Depressive Disorder Working Group, *VA/DoD Clinical Practice Guideline for Management of Major Depressive Disorder*, Washington, D.C.: U.S. Department of Veterans Affairs and U.S. Department of Defense, version 2.0, 2009. As of August 16, 2016:
http://www.healthquality.va.gov/mdd/MDD_FULL_3c1.pdf

———, *VA/DoD Clinical Practice Guideline for Management of Major Depressive Disorder*, Washington, D.C.: U.S. Department of Veterans Affairs and U.S. Department of Defense, version 3.0, April 2016. As of August 16, 2016:
http://www.healthquality.va.gov/guidelines/mh/mdd/index.asp

Management of Post-Traumatic Stress Working Group, *VA/DoD Clinical Practice Guideline for Management of Post-Traumatic Stress Disorder*, Washington, D.C.: U.S. Department of Veterans Affairs and U.S. Department of Defense, October 2010. As of August 16, 2016:
http://www.healthquality.va.gov/PTSD-full-2010c.pdf

Martsolf, Grant R., Karen Chan Osilla, Daniel Mandel, Kimberly A. Hepner, and Carrie M. Farmer, *Assessing the Quality and Value of Psychological Health Care in Civilian Health Plans: Lessons and Implications for the Military Health System*, Santa Monica, Calif.: RAND Corporation, RR-759-OSD, 2015. As of August 19, 2016:
http://www.rand.org/pubs/research_reports/RR759.html

Maslach, Christina, Susan E. Jackson, and Michael P. Leiter, *Maslach Burnout Inventory Manual*, 3rd ed., Palo Alto, Calif.: Consulting Psychologists Press, 1996.

Meredith, Lisa S., Lisa V. Rubenstein, Kathryn Rost, Daniel E. Ford, Nancy Gordon, Paul Nutting, Patti Camp, and Kenneth B. Wells, "Treating Depression in Staff-Model Versus Network-Model Managed Care Organizations," *Journal of General Internal Medicine*, Vol. 14, No. 1, January 1999, pp. 39–48.

Miliken, Charles S., Jennifer L. Auchterlonie, and Charles W. Hoge, "Longitudinal Assessment of Mental Health Problems Among Active and Reserve Component Soldiers Returning from the Iraq War," *JAMA*, Vol. 298, No. 18, November 14, 2007, pp. 2141–2148.

Morris, David W., and Madhukar H. Trivedi, "Measurement-Based Care for Unipolar Depression," *Current Psychiatry Reports*, Vol. 13, No. 6, December 2011, pp. 446–458.

Nacasch, Nitzah, Edna B. Foa, Jonathan D. Huppert, Dana Tzur, Leah Fostick, Yula Dinstein, Michael Polliack, and Joseph Zohar, "Prolonged Exposure Therapy for Combat- and Terror-Related Posttraumatic Stress Disorder: A Randomized Control Comparison with Treatment as Usual," *Journal of Clinical Psychiatry*, Vol. 72, No. 9, September 2011, pp. 1174–1180.

Naval Center for Combat and Operational Stress Control, "Behavioral Health Data Portal (BHDP)," undated(a). As of August 1, 2016:
http://www.med.navy.mil/sites/nmcsd/nccosc/technology/bhdp/index.aspx

———, "Psychological Health Pathways (PHP)," undated(b). As of August 1, 2016:
http://www.med.navy.mil/sites/nmcsd/nccosc/healthProfessionalsV2/psychologicalHealthPathways/Pages/default.aspx

Norcross, John C., and Jessica D. Rogan, "Psychologists Conducting Psychotherapy in 2012: Current Practices and Historical Trends Among Division 29 Members," *Psychotherapy*, Vol. 50, No. 4, December 2013, pp. 490–495.

Obama, Barack, "Executive Order—Improving Access to Mental Health Services for Veterans, Service Members, and Military Families," Washington, D.C.: White House, Office of the Press Secretary, August 31, 2012. As of September 14, 2016:
http://www.whitehouse.gov/the-press-office/2012/08/31/
executive-order-improving-access-mental-health-services-veterans-service

Office of Management and Budget, *Office of Management and Budget, Standards and Guidelines for Statistical Surveys*, Washington, D.C., September 2006. As of August 19, 2016:
http://www.whitehouse.gov/sites/default/files/omb/inforeg/statpolicy/standards_stat_surveys.pdf

Ogunfowora, Babatunde, and Martin Drapeau, "A Study of the Relationship Between Personality Traits and Theoretical Orientation Preferences," *Counselling and Psychotherapy Research*, Vol. 8, No. 3, September 2008, pp. 151–159.

Pingitore, David P., Richard M. Scheffler, Tetine Sentell, and Joyce C. West, "Comparison of Psychiatrists and Psychologists in Clinical Practice," *Psychiatric Services*, Vol. 53, No. 8, August 2002, pp. 977–983.

Powers, Mark B., Jacqueline M. Halpern, Michael P. Ferenschak, Seth J. Gillihan, and Edna B. Foa, "A Metaanalytic Review of Prolonged Exposure for Posttraumatic Stress Disorder," *Clinical Psychology Review*, Vol. 30, No. 6, August 2010, pp. 635–641.

Poznanski, Joseph J., and Jim McLennan, "Conceptualizing and Measuring Counselors' Theoretical Orientation," *Journal of Counseling Psychology*, Vol. 42, No. 4, October 1995, pp. 411–422.

Quaadgras, Anne, Amy Glasmeier, and Ken Kaplan, *Building a Better USMC Psychological Health System: Coordination Analysis and Design Recommendations*, Cambridge, Mass.: Sociotechnical Systems Research Center, Massachusetts Institute of Technology, 2016.

Ramchand, Rajeev, Benjamin R. Karney, Karen Chan Osilla, Rachel M. Burns, and Leah Barnes Caldarone, "Prevalence of PTSD, Depression, and TBI Among Returning Servicemembers," in Tanielian, Terri and Lisa H. Jaycox, eds., *Invisible Wounds of War: Psychological and Cognitive Injuries, Their Consequences, and Services to Assist Recovery*, Santa Monica, Calif.: RAND Corporation, MG-720-CCF, 2008, pp. 35–85. As of August 16, 2016:
http://www.rand.org/pubs/monographs/MG720.html

Ramchand, Rajeev, Rena Rudavsky, Sean Grant, Terri Tanielian, and Lisa Jaycox, "Prevalence of, Risk Factors for, and Consequences of Posttraumatic Stress Disorder and Other Mental Health Problems in Military Populations Deployed to Iraq and Afghanistan," *Current Psychiatry Reports*, Vol. 17, No. 5, May 2015.

Ramchand, Rajeev, Terry L. Schell, Benjamin R. Karney, Karen Chan Osilla, Rachel M. Burns, and Leah Barnes Caldarone, "Disparate Prevalence Estimates of PTSD Among Service Members Who Served in Iraq and Afghanistan: Possible Explanations," *Journal of Traumatic Stress*, Vol. 23, No. 1, February 2010, pp. 59–68.

Reardon, Maureen Lyons, Kelly C. Cukrowicz, Mark D. Reeves, and T. E. Joiner, "Duration and Regularity of Therapy Attendance as Predictors of Treatment Outcome in an Adult Outpatient Population," *Psychotherapy Research*, Vol. 12, No. 3, 2002, pp. 273–285.

Schell, Terry L., and Grant N. Marshall, "Survey of Individuals Previously Deployed for OEF/OIF," in Terri Tanielian and Lisa H. Jaycox, eds., *Invisible Wounds of War: Psychological and Cognitive Injuries, Their Consequences, and Services to Assist Recovery*, Santa Monica, Calif.: RAND Corporation, MG-720-CCF, 2008, pp. 87–115. As of August 16, 2016:
http://www.rand.org/pubs/monographs/MG720z1

Scott, Kelli, and Cara C. Lewis, "Using Measurement-Based Care to Enhance Any Treatment," *Cognitive and Behavioral Practice*, Vol. 22, No. 1, February 2015, pp. 49–59.

Shin, Hana J., Mark A. Greenbaum, Shaili Jain, and Craig S. Rosen, "Associations of Psychotherapy Dose and SSRI or SNRI Refills with Mental Health Outcomes Among Veterans with PTSD," *Psychiatric Services*, Vol. 65, No. 10, October 2014, pp. 1244–1248. As of February 15, 2017:
http://www.ncbi.nlm.nih.gov/pubmed/24981643

Sholomskas, Diane E., Gia Syracuse-Siewert, Bruce J. Rounsaville, Samuel A. Ball, Kathryn F. Nuro, and Kathleen M. Carroll, "We Don't Train in Vain: A Dissemination Trial of Three Strategies of Training Clinicians in Cognitive-Behavioral Therapy," *Journal of Consulting and Clinical Psychology*, Vol. 73, No. 1, February 2005, pp. 106–115.

Smith, Tyler C., Mark Zamorski, Besa Smith, James R. Riddle, Cynthia A. LeardMann, Timothy S. Wells, Charles C. Engel, Charles W. Hoge, Joyce Adkins, and Dan Blaze, "The Physical and Mental Health of a Large Military Cohort: Baseline Functional Health Status of the Millennium Cohort," *BMC Public Health*, Vol. 7, No. 1, 2007.

Stein, Dan J., Jonathan C. Ipser, and Soraya Seedat, "Pharmacotherapy for Post Traumatic Stress Disorder (PTSD)," *Cochrane Database of Systematic Reviews*, No. 1, January 2009.

Tanielian, Terri, Mahlet A. Woldetsadik, Lisa H. Jaycox, Caroline Batka, Shaela Moen, Carrie Farmer, and Charles C. Engel, "Barriers to Engaging Service Members in Mental Health Care Within the U.S. Military Health System," *Psychiatric Services*, Vol. 67, No. 7, July 2016, pp. 718–727.

Trangle, Michael, J. Gursky, R. Haight, J. Hardwig, T. Hinnenkamp, D. Kessler, N. Mack, and M. Myszkowshi, *Health Care Guideline: Depression in Primary Care*, Institute for Clinical Systems Improvement, March 2016.

U.S. Department of the Air Force, *Air Force Instruction 44-172*, Operations, Medical, AF/SG3/5, 2015.
http://static.e-publishing.af.mil/production/1/af_sg/publication/afi44-172/afi44-172.pdf

U.S. Government Accountability Office, *Defense Health Care: Additional Information Needed About Mental Health Provider Staffing Needs*, Washington, D.C.: GAO-15-55, January 30, 2015.

———, *Defense Health Care: DOD Is Meeting Most Mental Health Care Access Standards, but It Needs a Standard for Follow-Up Appointments*, Washington, D.C.: GAO-16-416, April 28, 2016.

Uniformed Services University, 2016. As of October 31, 2016:
https://www.usuhs.edu/

VanGeest, Jonathan B., Timothy P. Johnson, and Verna L. Welch, "Methodologies for Improving Response Rates in Surveys of Physicians: A Systematic Review," *Evaluation and the Health Professions*, Vol. 30, No. 4, December 2007, pp. 303–321.

Weinick, Robin M., Ellen Burke Beckjord, Carrie M. Farmer, Laurie T. Martin, Emily M. Gillen, Joie D. Acosta, Michael P. Fisher, Jeffrey Garnett, Gabriella C. Gonzalez, Todd C. Helmus, Lisa H. Jaycox, Kerry Reynolds, Nicholas Salcedo, and Deborah M. Scharf, *Programs Addressing Psychological Health and Traumatic Brain Injury Among U.S. Military Servicemembers and Their Families*, Santa Monica, Calif.: RAND Corporation, TR-950-OSD, 2011. As of August 16, 2016:
http://www.rand.org/pubs/technical_reports/TR950.html

Wells, Timothy S., Shannon C. Miller, Amy B. Adler, Charles C. Engel, Tyler C. Smith, and John A. Fairbank, "Mental Health Impact of the Iraq and Afghanistan Conflicts: A Review of US Research, Service Provision, and Programmatic Responses," *International Review of Psychiatry*, Vol. 23, No. 2, April 2011, pp. 144–152.

Wilk, Joshua E., Joyce C. West, Farifteh F. Duffy, Richard K. Herrell, Donald S. Rae, and Charles W. Hoge, "Use of Evidence-Based Treatment for Posttraumatic Stress Disorder in Army Behavioral Healthcare," *Psychiatry*, Vol. 76, No. 4, Winter 2013, pp. 336–348.

Woodson, Jonathan, Assistant Secretary of Defense for Health Affairs, *Military Treatment Facility Mental Health Clinical Outcomes Guidance*, memorandum, September 9, 2013. As of August 19, 2016:
http://www.dcoe.mil/Libraries/Documents/MentalHealthClinicalOutcomesGuidance_Woodson.pdf